THE

ultimate

guide TO

chakras

The Beginner's Guide
to Balancing, Healing, and
Unblocking Your Chakras for
Health and Positive Energy

Athena Perrakis, Ph.D.

FAIR WINDS

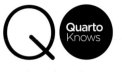

Brimming with creative inspiration, how-to projects, and useful information to enrich your everyday life, Quarto Knows is a favorite destination for those pursuing their interests and passions. Visit our site and dig deeper with our books into your area of interest: Quarto Creates, Quarto Cooks, Quarto Homes, Quarto Lives, Quarto Drives, Quarto Explores, Quarto Gifts, or Quarto Kids.

© 2018 Quarto Publishing Group USA Inc.
Text © 2018 Athena Perrakis
Photography © 2018 Sage Goddess
Illustration © 2018 Roberta Orpwood

First Published in 2018 by Fair Winds Press, an imprint of The Quarto Group,
100 Cummings Center, Suite 265-D, Beverly, MA 01915, USA.
T (978) 282-9590 F (978) 283-2742 QuartoKnows.com

Fair Winds Press titles are also available at discount for retail, wholesale, promotional, and bulk purchase. For details, contact the Special Sales Manager by email at specialsales@quarto.com or by mail at The Quarto Group, Attn: Special Sales Manager, 100 Cummings Center Suite 265D, Beverly, MA 01915 USA.

22 21 20 19   5

ISBN: 978-1-59233-847-4

Digital edition published in 2018
eISBN: 978-1-63159-537-0

Library of Congress Cataloging-in-Publication Data

Perrakis, Athena, author.
The ultimate guide to chakras : the beginner's guide to balancing,
    healing, and unblocking your chakras for health and positive energy /
    Athena Perrakis, Ph.D.
ISBN   9781631595370 (e-book) | ISBN 9781592338474 (pbk.)
1. Energy medicine--Popular works. 2. Chakras--Health
    aspects--Popular works. 3. Self-care, Health--Popular works.
LCC RZ421 (ebook) | LCC RZ421 .P47 2018 (print)
DDC   615.8/52--dc23
2018012264 (print) | 2018014850 (ebook)

Design: Tanya Naylor, tanyasoffice.com
Page Layout: Tanya Naylor, tanyasoffice.com
Photography: Sage Goddess
Illustration: Roberta Orpwood

Printed in China

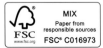

I dedicate this book to my husband and soulmate David and our children, Nick and Zoe; my parents, Nick and Marie; BrookeLynn, my twin spirit; my brother, Jeff; my sister, Kristin; my good friends, Patty and Leo; my grandmothers, Pearl and Fotini; and all members of the Magical Sabbatical. I am because we are and they were. A'ho.

Contents

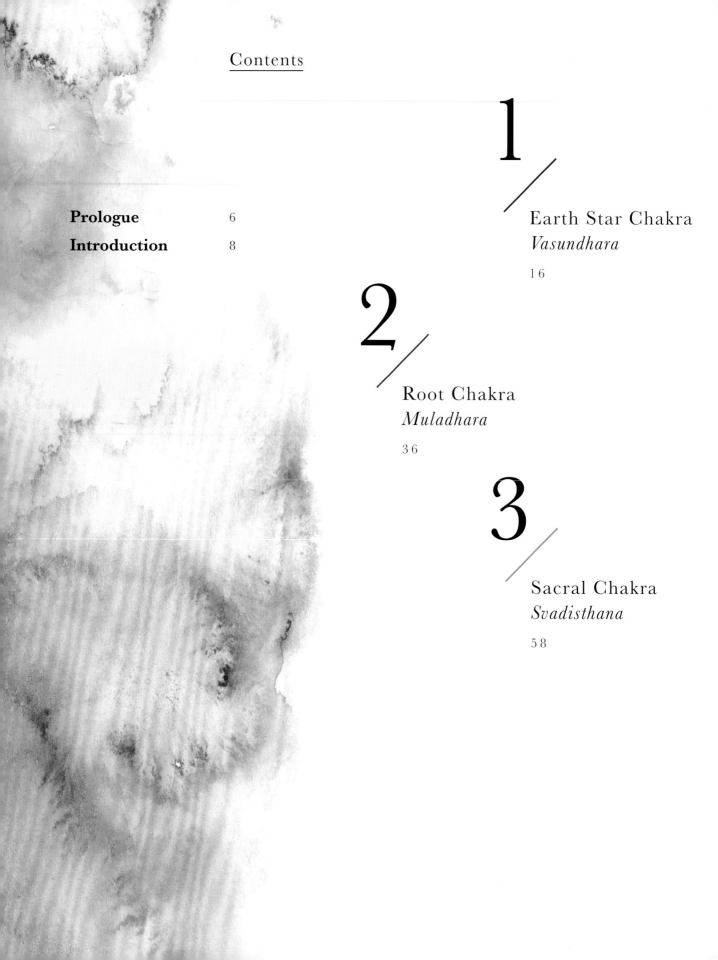

Prologue

Much of today's accepted metaphysical wisdom has deep roots and long lineages dating back to early civilizations and ancient cultures. When you trace these roots back to their source, incredible doors of awareness open to you, because these connections to history, mythology, geology, archaeology, and etymologies of ancient languages are what keep this wisdom alive. When you are mindful and reverent of the past, you both honor your ancestors and do a great service to your lineage.

The purpose of this book, then, is to teach you about the chakras, or energy centers, found within and adjacent to the human body. In Sanskrit, arguably the oldest and most sacred living language, chakra means "wheel." This translation hints at the spinning, circular movement of each energy center, which simultaneously receives and sends information to and from you all the time.

But why are chakras so important, and why have they been a focus of spiritual teaching since ancient times? The answer is simple: Chakras, or energy centers, are the gathering places of energy within and adjacent to your physical body. It is important to study them because they are your body's energy vortexes; they determine where, how, and for what purpose energy is flowing within your physical body and your etheric body (that is, the first layer of the aura or human energy field).

Energy flow is vitally important. It dictates your health, happiness, and whether you are in harmony with your environment. That's why understanding your chakras and improving energy flow through them can literally bring you greater health, happiness, harmony, prosperity, love, wellness, protection, and comfort. Your chakras are doorways to spiritual power and possibility, and as such have been an ongoing source of fascination and study for thousands of years. What's more, each one of your chakras contains an ancient key that can unlock solutions to modern challenges and dilemmas. This means that you are about to learn secrets that were once known only to our ancestors, and to bring those traditions into present time.

The origins of the modern chakra system can be traced back to the Vedas, the oldest and most sacred texts of ancient Indian culture. The Vedas are a body of what is known as knowledge texts written in Sanskrit and are the foundation of modern Ayurvedic medicine and Hindu wisdom. Hindus consider the Vedas to be supernaturally authored texts full of channeled messages designed to guide and help humans as they evolve. There are four Vedas, and each has been classified into four text types. Of all of the Vedas, the Upanashads are most widely known and recognized, and in Sanskrit, *upanashad* translates literally to "sitting down close to," which refers to the way in which students gather close to their teacher in order to receive spiritual information and wisdom. The Upanashads—or Vedanta, one of the Vedic classifications—contain all of the Vedic wisdom regarding spirituality and meditation. In addition to information about the chakras, they also contain central Hindu concepts of God (Brahman) and the Soul (Atman) plus the foundations of modern Hindu practice that also have echoes in Buddhism and Sikhism.

Thus the chakra system is a mainstay of spiritual practices around the world (including yoga). It includes seven primary physical energy centers as well as two additional anchor energy centers that connect you to Earth and Spirit. However, some traditions point to 50 to 108 energy centers in the body and aura that correspond to letters of the Sanskrit alphabet and call for the recitation of Sanskrit mantras or prayers. This phenomenon of multiple energy centers aligned with the ancient Sanskrit language forms the basis of modern mantra recitation practices, whereby reciting a sacred Sanskrit mantra 108 times is said to activate the 108 energy centers of the body.

However, this book's focus is the basic physical chakra system and the two anchor chakras, including their gemstones, essential oils, tarot, and astrological, mythological, and historical correspondences. This is because the seven primary chakras are the most widely agreed-upon energy centers across all spiritual traditions that acknowledge the flow of energy through the human body. Beyond these seven, two additional chakras are needed to anchor the flow of energy back into the planet and back up to spirit—that is, a return to Source or to a Higher Power—and so a total of nine are explored here in depth. As you read this book, allow yourself to feel the words and to receive them at the specific energy center to which they refer. Where possible, you might even consider placing your hand over the relevant energy center as you explore the pages dedicated to it, since chakras are vortex points of coagulated energy that can only be partially understood on an intellectual level. As you'll see, the rest of the experience is highly emotional, intuitive, and experiential.

To that end, each chapter includes a specific meditation and mantra for each chakra based on the ancient Vedic texts so that you can practice working with the chakras in physical, intellectual, and spiritual ways. Connecting with the chakras in multiple

ways allows them to make themselves known to you on a deeper level. After all, spiritual teachings are not meant to be entirely intellectual exercises; you are meant to live into the ideas, experience the concepts, and see the inherent beauty they represent.

The nine chakras explored in this book begin beneath your feet, with your most grounded and powerful connection to Earth: the Earth Star Chakra, which is referred to as *Vasundhara* (Sanskrit for "daughter of the Earth"). Then, the Base, or Root, Chakra (*Muladhara*) is followed by the Sacral Chakra (*Svadhisthana*); the Solar Plexus Chakra (*Manipura*); the Heart Chakra (*Anahata*); the Throat Chakra (*Vishuddha*); the Third Eye Chakra (*Ajna*); the Crown Chakra (*Sahasrara*); and, finally, the Soul Star Chakra, which is referred to as *Sutara* in Sanskrit or "Holy Star." Following this order, the book will unfold from Earth to Sky, from physical human reality toward your uppermost point of access to Source energy and creation. The journey skyward will be echoed within your own spirit, and as you read, you will find that your body feels more aligned and comfortable, that your soul feels more peaceful and calm, and that your mind feels enchanted, relaxed, and excited to explore the limits of this new framework.

Think of yourself, then, as the Fool from the major arcana of the tarot as you step into these pages. You are ready to embark on a new adventure that you know will transform you—and you are aware that this transformation is necessary, even critical, to your development. I advise you to read this book slowly, allowing the words to move through you and into you, settling deep into the groundwater of your experience and your desire to expand. As you work through the various Embodiment Exercises, you will experience a renewed connection to the energies located in each chakra and will begin to embody them more significantly in your life and spiritual practice.

Soon, when a challenge arises, or when someone in your life is in need of healing, you will have an immediate sense of which chakras need to be incorporated into your healing work. You will know how to work with the energies to assess, evaluate, and activate your chakras in order to improve your own well-being, the well-being of others, and the planet as a whole.

Introduction:
What Is a Chakra?

While chakras have become a popular metaphysical topic of discussion and subject of study, the concept of the chakras is nothing new. But first of all, what is a chakra? The word *chakra* comes from the Sanskrit word for "wheel" or "disk," and, as part of ancient Vedic healing practices and techniques—many of which endure today—yogis have worked with the chakra system for thousands of years. That's because in Ayurvedic medicine, illness is seen as an energy blockage anchored in one or more of the chakras. Other healing modalities, such as acupuncture, also acknowledge the blocked flow of energy as a root cause of disease and pain. In fact, Western allopathic medicine is one of the few traditions that does *not* locate energy blockages in order to alleviate pain and suffering in the body, mind, and spirit.

Perhaps you're asking yourself why energy moves through disks, or chakras, in the first place. Let me explain: In the yogic tradition, *prana*, or life force energy, is by design and necessity a flowing source of God/Source/Creator consciousness. Energy is always flowing, and this is a fact: Quantum mechanics has proved, via zero-point theory, that particles are never at rest; even in a resting state, there will always be non-zero kinetic energy. And since all matter is energy, even when you are physically at rest, you are in constant motion on a subatomic level. Beyond your physical body, you have an etheric, or "subtle," body that remains at a higher vibratory state and thus is not visible to the eye. That subtle body is home to your chakras, or energy centers, where energy naturally coagulates at nine central points from just above your head to just under your feet.

Most people are aware that their physical well-being is much more than a physical issue, so it's not hard to understand and appreciate the idea of energy centers that are open and functioning well, freely, and comfortably, as opposed to energy centers that are closed, constricted, and uncomfortable. Since pain is nothing more than data being processed over the wires of your central nervous system—information designed to tell you that a system is offline or awry—it is easy to see how pain begins energetically in one of the chakras and, from there, starts to manifest in the physical body, often in close proximity to the chakra origin of the energy wound or trauma. Western medicine treats the symptoms of energy issues, which is so helpful: Where would many of us be without the ability to manage pain and symptomatic suffering? But in order to reach the source or root cause of your physical dis-ease, it is wise to look deeper, and sometimes further back, than ever before—back into your maternal and paternal lines, since many of your current energy patterns were inherited from the ancestors who came before you.

For example, experiences of war in your genetic line can manifest as Root Chakra imbalances around safety. You may not inherit the physical experience of war, but you can inherit the energy imprint of it. If you wonder why you came into this life feeling unsafe and unable to rest, you may not have a single physical symptom—but your feelings may indicate that something is off balance. If you can address these feelings, which precede physical pain and disease, much healing can be accomplished.

This process begins in the chakra system. Once you identify the chakra of origin for any of your current challenges, you can establish a plan to shift and move the energy, allowing the chakra to function normally and realigning it once again with the other energy centers. From there, physical healing—which may seem to be a spontaneous miracle, but is actually rooted in alchemical transformation from within—can begin to unfold. Your entire life can change. It all begins with knowledge and making the choice to say yes to a new way of thinking about your life, your health, and your happiness.

Embodiment Exercise:
Sensing Ancestral Imprints

In this exercise, you will receive guidance about where you need to integrate ancestral wisdom in your life today. Ancestral wisdom can take two forms: wisdom from your material ancestors in this lifetime (your mothers, grandmothers, fathers, and grandfathers); and wisdom from your spirit ancestors, i.e., those who share your expansive spiritual lineage. Your soul has traveled many places across many lifetimes, and your many physical bodies from those lifetimes gathered cumulative wisdom that sits within your spirit's wisdom archives.

Take a moment to sit comfortably and relax your shoulders, calling your energy into present time from wherever it may be, whoever it might be with. Do this by speaking your name out loud, over and over, in a soft voice or by imagining your name written into sand on a beautiful beach. Then let this meditation guide you.

1/ Gently coming into this moment, notice your fingers and toes, giving thanks for your breath, becoming aware of your heartbeat as an echo of the Divine, and calming your entire central nervous system.

2/ Call to mind an image of your father or grandfather, whichever is easiest for you. (If you never had a father figure in your life, ask your guides to connect you with your male next-of-kin in the spirit realm.) Notice where in your body you feel a connection to the Paternal Line, the male beings of light and energy from whom you physically descend. Since the left side of the body governs the masculine and paternal energy streams, you are most likely to sense male energy there. Perhaps your left hand will tingle or feel warm. Stretch out your left arm and imagine sending a bright beam of light to receive and send information related to your male line. Take note of any pleasant or uncomfortable feelings. You do not need to fix or adjust them—simply notice them. Send those thoughts and feelings love, and let them go.

3/ Next, call to mind an image of your mother or grandmother, whichever is easiest for you. (If you never had a mother figure in your life, ask your guides to connect you with your female next-of-kin in the spirit realm.) Notice where in your body you feel a connection to the Maternal Line, the female beings of light and energy from whom you physically descend. Just as the left side of the body governs the paternal energy stream, so the right side governs the feminine, maternal energy streams. You are most likely to sense female energy on the right side of the body, especially in the palms of your hands, the top of your head, and the soles of your feet—the three primary places in the body where energy is stored and easily released. Take note of any pleasant or uncomfortable feelings. Send them love, and let them go.

4/ Now, bring your awareness to those places in your body (or mind or spirit) where discomfort arose. Notice without judgment whether those places align to the chakras, or energy centers. If you sense discomfort at the top of your head, for example, that pain might represent an ancestral imprint related to spiritual development. Perhaps the wisdom you need to access and integrate right now in your life is related to a spiritual matter or practice, so pay closer attention than normal to spiritual aspects of your life.

5/ Then, bring your awareness to those places in your body, mind, or spirit where pleasant feelings arose. Notice also without judgment whether those places align to the chakras, or energy centers. If you sense discomfort at the base of your spine, for example, that pain might represent an ancestral imprint related to your safety or home. Pay closer attention than usual to matters related to these subjects.

6/ As you explore the chapters ahead, let this information guide the way you engage with and prioritize what you read, and at what pace, so that you can receive the healing you need in this moment, knowing that your energy needs may shift and change over time. It is ever a process, always unfolding. Amen, A'ho, So it is.

How Does Energy Move?

We know that energy moves because it is a coagulation of quantum particles that are never at rest—but how does it move? Energy (or *prana* or *chi*) flows through a central channel or column of light called the *Sushumna*, which means "gracious" or "kind" in Sanskrit. All seven of the corporal chakras (meaning those attached to the human body) reside in the Sushumna; the secondary chakras discussed in this book, specifically the Earth Star and Soul Star chakras, flow above and below the Sushumna.

There are two energy lines called the *nadi*, one masculine and one feminine, that wrap around the Sushumna in a DNA-like spiral of light, crossing at the *Muladhara* or Root Chakra, *Manipura* or Solar Plexus Chakra, *Vissudha* or Throat Chakra, and *Sahasrara* or Crown Chakra. At each of these energy centers the masculine and feminine lines cross and merge. (Interestingly, the energy centers where the lines do not merge represent natural points of integration of masculine and feminine. This is true for the Sacral Chakra, or point of conception of life; the Heart Chakra, or point of conception of love; and the Third Eye Chakra, or point of conception of wisdom.) Just as your central nervous system regulates and manages all messages within your physical body, so your chakra system regulates and manages all messages within your subtle, or etheric, body.

Three Steps to Balancing the Chakras for Optimal Function

If illness begins in the body as blocked energy, then the optimal function of the chakras—and the optimal flow of energy through and between them—is critical to health. But how do you know whether your chakras are balanced? And if they are out of balance or blocked, how do you regain equilibrium and flow? That's what this book is all about. In each of the chapters that follow, you will find specific tips and techniques for aligning each individual chakra. First, here are three steps for assessing, aligning, and activating the energy flow throughout the chakra system. Follow these steps anytime you feel sluggish, sad, or unable to sleep through the night; those are three common signs of chakra imbalance that can be easily corrected, and once corrected, can be easily maintained.

Please, never take this guidance, or anyone else's, above your own. Trust your inner knowing and your senses. They will always lead you to the right path at the right time. Take and use what feels accurate here for you, and leave the rest.

Step 1: Assessing Energy Flow

When you feel sadder, more agitated, or more tired than usual, or when you feel increased pain or discomfort in your body, it is time to assess your personal energy flow (PEF). Your PEF governs how you feel every day, and is affected by both internal and external factors. By simply reading this book, you are becoming consciously aware of your PEF, which is a critical first step in the assessment process. Once you know what flow feels like, your body can record a memory of this state of being and can then regulate itself back to that state of flow, or balance, when energy waxes or wanes.

Remember that the human body is a magnificently intelligent system. You can trust your body to heal itself in every moment; in fact, your body wants nothing more than to reach a state of homeostasis, or perfect balance. Just like every organ in your body works to reach and maintain homeostasis, because balance is the comfort zone of the universe, so, too, do your energy centers work together intelligently to create harmonious balance within your system.

That's right: Balance is your birthright.

You move away from balance consciously, by practicing extremes in your ways of eating, moving, and working with energies in your primary energy field. For instance, eating too much food, or not enough of it, can throw the physical system off balance, since food is energy. Moving too much, or not enough, can also impact the way energy flows in your body. And too much stress, sorrow, tension, chatter, and noise can pull you off course energetically and separate you from your peace, from your center, and from your connection to Source. None of this happens overnight, though; these events unfold slowly, over decades of not paying close enough attention to staying balanced.

Embodiment Exercise: Chakra Assessment

Just as your physical body benefits from a regular checkup, your chakras also benefit from regular assessment. There are many different ways to evaluate the condition of the chakras, but this exercise is one easy way to quickly and effectively evaluate the current condition of your energy centers, as well as receive guidance and wisdom about where your attention is needed now.

Take a moment to call your energy into present time by speaking your name out loud, over and over, in a soft voice, or by imagining your name written into sand on a beautiful beach. Invite your guides to be present with you. Call in the guardians of space and time to anchor the four corners and four cardinal elements as you begin a scan of your sacred energy centers.

Begin in the East when you call upon guardian energies. You can do this by speaking the following words out loud or whispering them softly to yourself: "Guardian Keepers of the East, energies of air and flight, we welcome you. Please bring us a bright new beginning and new wisdom to help us integrate our work. Guardian Keepers of the South, energies of fire and power, we welcome you. Please bring us a strong and courageous spirit to empower our work. Guardian Keepers of the West, energies of water and flow, we welcome you. Please purify us and cleanse our hearts as we bring love to the world, and please open a container for prosperity to flow freely toward our work. Guardian Keepers of the North, energies of Earth and time, we welcome you. Please ground and protect us as we embody our work. We thank you for your presence. Amen, A'ho, So it is." Then let this meditation guide you.

1/ First, notice every part of your body, giving thanks as you go. Thank the soles of your feet, and the Earth below you, for rooting you into the present moment and reminding you of your inherent safety and sovereignty. Thank your legs and hips, your lower back and pelvic floor, for guiding you and inspiring you, and for bringing the force of creation and life through you. Thank your ovaries or testes, your life-giving capacity and birthing potential, your sensual self. Thank your digestive system and kidneys; thank your adrenal system, your lungs, your breath of life. Thank your heart and your esophagus, your throat, tongue, and teeth. Thank your voice and your truth. Thank your face and your cheeks, your seeing eyes and your knowing eye. Thank your ears and the top of your head, your hair, and the soft spot of knowing that connects you to your Creator.

2/ Thank your body as a whole, just as it is. Allow all to be, just as it is, right here, right now, as it desires to be. There is nothing to change, nothing to fix. All is available for noticing, for scanning, for discerning.

3/ Then, speak these words aloud: "Energy centers, reveal your needs. Speak your truths to me. Show me where my attention is needed so that I may invoke the healing potential of my own intelligent system. I trust in my own ability to restore, recover, and repair anything that needs it, in perfect time and alignment with my whole health. Amen, A'ho, So it is."

Notice what comes forward for you in this exercise, and pay attention to even the subtlest of signs. You might see something, sense something, smell something, feel something. All information is welcome. Then journal what you have noticed, and make a note of the date and time.

Continue to record any thoughts, feelings, or emotions that arise in the next forty-eight hours. If you feel called to work with sound, crystals or gemstones, essential oils, herbs, light, massage, Reiki, or other healing methods or modalities, heed the call. (If you are a practiced healer, do this in your usual way.) In this way, you can use your intuition to pursue what your physical and etheric bodies need at this time.

You will learn about the gemstone, essential oil, and herbal correspondences for each chakra in this book. When working with herbs, you can choose to use them in either their raw herbal or distilled essential oil form. Both are powerful. Choose the form you work with based on what is available locally to you where you live and what resonates most deeply. For example, with dried herbs, you can make incenses and sacred bundles to burn. With essential oils, you can create perfumes and body products. We list herbs aligned to each chakra.

The more time you spend observing your chakras and energy centers, coming into more profound awareness of the signs and messages around you, the more you will become familiar with changes in the subtle systems and be able to respond to them before they manifest in physical challenges or symptoms. This, ultimately, is what it means to be a healer. You might also consider the possibility that your intuition is always guiding you to attune yourself to the health and vitality of your chakras. Although your chakras operate synchronistically and without need for your direct intervention, your intuition can and will often guide you to direct your attention to a particular chakra when its energies are needed or activated in your energy field.

Step 2: Aligning Energy Flow

Once you have assessed your current state of energy flow, noticing pain or resistance in particular areas, you can work on a specific chakra (or multiple chakras) to bring each center into balance before aligning the entire system for optimal flow. Aligning your system can be done using visualization, crystal therapy, essential oils via anointing rituals, or all three methods. Taking an integrated approach is best when healing and aligning chakras, so if you have access to gemstones and essential oils, by all means integrate them into your practice. Each tool offers a frequency, or vibration, and employs a different energy stream to bring its healing to the chakra, or energy center.

Over time, you can isolate your work with these tools to determine what works best for you and when, where, and how. This is when your intuition will begin to play a very significant role in your spiritual development and overall healing. In the process of healing yourself and achieving balance and wellness, you will learn what your soul gifts are (if you have not downloaded this wisdom already!) and in so doing, you will become the healer you were born to be in this lifetime.

Embodiment Exercise:
Weaving the Thread of Healing

In so many ways, healing is alignment; healing requires all systems to hang in a sacred balance. In this exercise, you will experience alignment via the most beautiful connection among your chakras, gently tethering them to the Earth below and the realms above with a golden thread of light and magic.

Before you begin, take a moment to call your energy into present time by speaking your name out loud, over and over, in a soft voice, or by imagining your name written into sand on a beautiful beach. Then, move into this meditation:

1/ To align the chakras, begin by visualizing a golden thread of light threaded through a beautiful golden needle of intention. What intention will you imprint upon your golden needle as you use it to weave the golden thread of light through your energy centers? You can choose healing, happiness, love, prosperity, balance, joy, peace, or whatever resonates with you.

2/ Once you have centered your focus on your intention for your needle, see the golden thread passing through the eye, and then wrap the golden thread of light around your Earth Star Chakra, which pulsates just beneath your feet, as an anchor between you and the Earth. Pull the thread up and gently wrap it around your Root Chakra, calling in your intention for grounding and protection. Then, pull the golden thread up

and around your Sacral Chakra, calling in your intention for creativity and procreativity, sensuality, sexuality, and passion. Imagine a well of passion and desire pulsing within you, all of your desires and longings made manifest in a state of sacred intimacy and pleasure.

3/ From there, gently wrap the golden thread around the Sacral Chakra before threading it up toward your Solar Plexus Chakra as you set an intention for personal power and possibility. Imagine the deepest sense of self-esteem and self-worth enveloping you as you pull the thread up toward your Heart Chakra, winding it around your heart in alignment with your intention for love and divine union.

4/ As you weave the thread higher toward your Throat Chakra, you locate your center of Truth and anchor of Integrity, the bridge between who you are and how you present in the world. Wrapping the golden thread around your throat chakra now, imagine easy access to your full and unencumbered truth, yielding to the voice of your Highest Self and the voices of your guides as they seek to bring your closer to who you truly are.

5/ Now, as you wind the golden thread toward the upper chakras—first around your Third Eye Chakra, to access intuition and inner knowing, and then around your Crown Chakra, to deepen your connection to God/Source/Creator—you encounter a well of peace and a frequency of total alignment. Suddenly, all seems to be unfolding with grace, speaking to you of a wisdom that surpasses any human understanding. This frequency frees you to surrender your need to know, fix, or change anything about the present moment.

6/ In that place of peace, joy, and acceptance, you begin to gather the golden thread and wind it around the final chakra, the Soul Star Chakra, located approximately 12 inches (30 cm) above the top of the head. Once you have connected the thread to this uppermost point, the work of integrating all chakra energies is complete. You return to a state of balanced bliss without having to try or focus; you simply exist in a place of allowance and surrender, where healing begins and consciousness expands, connecting you to all that has ever been or ever will be. It is all here, and welcome, now in this moment and always. Amen, A'ho, So it is.

What a welcome moment. This is a chance to step fully into a state of active allowing, which is not only optimal for healing and balancing your energy centers, but is also the ideal energy container for manifestation. (Manifestation means many things to many people, but a spiritual definition of "manifestation" is the intentional transformation of thought into matter. In other words, manifestation is a wish come true.) The softer you can become and the more you can move out of your own way, the more easily you can see the things you desire unfold before you—almost effortlessly.

There is just one final step to the process of balancing energy flow in your body, and in many ways, it is the most important step of the three.

Step 3: Activating Energy Flow

Energy is present around you all of the time, but much of the energy surrounding you is dormant, awaiting activation. Certain energies cannot be activated at certain times; this depends on your personal state of spiritual development and which energies are considered valuable or important to your development by your spirit guides and higher self. All forces of nature are energy streams—think of love, healing, growth, balance. (Magic itself is an energy stream.) You will always be able to access the energies and sources of wisdom you need when you need them. If you find yourself unable to access or activate a particular energy stream, it simply means that you do not need it at this time.

Energy activation applies to all energies, even those in crystals and gemstones. Energy does not need your permission or activation to flow, but it does move more powerfully once activated. While energy activation is not the focus of this book, it is worthwhile to consider ways to improve energy flow via activation techniques so that you can experience an enhanced flow in your own body and facilitate a faster, deeper awakening of the energy centers in your body, which is critical for physical well-being.

Embodiment Exercise: Activating Energy Flow

To activate energy flow in your body, give permission to your spirit guides and higher self to access, open, and activate each chakra. This short meditation guides you to do just that.

1/ Begin by opening the central chakra chamber, or Sushumna, which is like a tube of light. Unscrew the bottom of the chamber beneath your feet, turning it to the right to open it, and then unscrew the top of the chamber above your head, again turning the top of the chamber to the right. Once you open the central chamber from the deepest roots below your feet to the highest clouds above you, you open the chakra system for assessment and alignment.

2/ Visualize your Earth Star and Root chakras opening, connecting you with and rooting you into the soil of Earth herself. Use the mantra "access, open, activate" as a touchstone phrase you repeat to yourself each time you visualize one of your chakras.

3/ Next, imagine your receiving chakras—Sacral, Solar Plexus, and Heart—opening to you, turning slowly and revealing their medicine of love and empowerment. Take a deep breath and repeat your mantra: "Access, open, activate." Then, imagine your projecting chakras—Throat, Third Eye, Crown, and Soul Star—revealing themselves to you, offering their medicine of wisdom, communication, and connection to the outer cosmic realms.

4/ Take a final breath and repeat the mantra one final time: "Access, open, activate." Once all chakras are accessed, opened, and activated, give thanks for this access and alignment. Then, close the Sushumna chamber, turning both top and bottom of the column to the left, sealing the chakras and returning your system to its waking, closed state.

You can choose to balance your chakras as often as you like. In my experience, this is not necessarily a daily or even a weekly practice: You should let your intuition guide you. If you notice that you feel less responsive, aligned, or energetic in your life, or that you lack the strength and tenacity you need to follow your dreams, your chakras may need attention and activation. Each time you engage in this process you will learn new ways to communicate with the energy flowing through your body, becoming increasingly aware and intuitively connected to your own needs in every moment.

As you continue on your path and deepen this practice, you may find that you don't need to continually clear the chakras or energy centers as often. That's because activating them consistently facilitates a self-clearing and self-managing process whereby the centers themselves, through their own intelligence and synergistic relationship with each other, can naturally restore their own balance without your explicit action or intervention. All systems in nature are guided by an inherently intuitive design and, as humans, we should avoid the presumption that the only way to "fix" or "improve" anything—including energy—is through our actions and intentions. In time, all energies needed for your physical, spiritual, and emotional well-being will become activated in your lifetimes. When you intervene, all you do is expedite what is already intended. Begin to trust that all forms of consciousness are expressing themselves fully and perfectly in this moment, including yourself.

Now that you have learned about the system of the chakras, including techniques for maintaining balance and flow among them, we'll turn to a deeper exploration of each individual energy center. Each is a microcosm of wisdom and meaning that regulates and aligns to specific energies in your physical and subtle bodies. In this nine-chakra model, the central chakras are the Heart and the Throat (Anahata and Vishuddha). The lower chakras, Earth Star to Solar Plexus, align to the Divine Feminine and are considered receptive chakras, where life force energy is received, channeled, processed, and grounded. The central chakras, Heart and Throat, align to Cosmic Love and Truth frequencies, and represent the integration of masculine and feminine energies. The upper chakras, Third Eye to Soul Star, align to the Divine Masculine and are considered projective chakras, where life force energy is filtered, translated, and then transmitted. As you explore each chakra, allow it to make itself known to you. Learning about chakras should be an intellectual, energetic, and somatic experience. A world of healing and beauty awaits, and it is my hope that you will be blessed by this wisdom.

In the chapters to come, through rich imagery and evocative descriptions, each chakra will reveal its piece of the Great Mystery to you. To that end, this book starts, as all good stories (and lessons) do, at the beginning; in the ground beneath your feet. We'll begin with the Earth Star, your homing device and your beacon of safety.

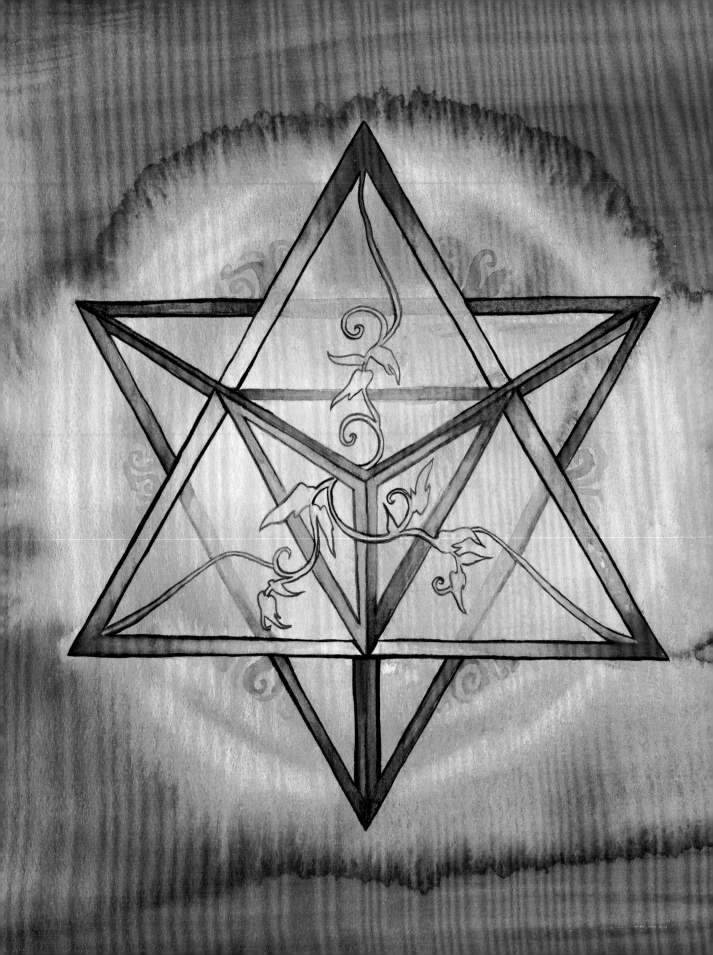

Ch

1

Earth Star Chakra—
Vasundhara

The Earth Star Chakra sits about 12 inches (30 cm) below your feet. It is a spinning wheel of light that connects you to Mother Earth, as well as all of the bones of the ancestors, the gem and mineral people (the spirits living within our gemstone and mineral tools), the faerie folk, and the collective consciousness of all humankind. For all of these reasons, many people feel that the Earth Star Chakra is the most important of the central nine energy centers.

Connecting to the Earth Star, or *Vasundhara*, allows you to ground and root our collective energy more firmly into Gaia's mortal matrix. Mother Gaia is the mother of all life on planet Earth, the keeper of ancient and grounded feminine wisdom. The Sanskrit name *Vasundhara* literally translates to "daughter of the Earth." Thus, this energy center is your oldest spiritual home. The Earth Star is also the Lower World of Shamanism, the entry point to a labyrinth of time, rock, and stone that leads to the molten core of our planet. What follows is a guided journey to help you explore the many aspects of this sacred birthplace.

Embodiment Exercise:
Earth Star Chakra Induction

Call your energy gently into present time by speaking your name out loud, over and over, in a soft voice, or by imagining your name written into sand on a beautiful beach. Your energy is the most powerful resonant tool you can use: Speaking it out loud or imagining it written brings your personal energy and focus into the present.

Bring your attention to this moment. Here begins a journey to encounter the Earth Star Chakra—your closest energy connection to Mother Gaia herself, and the part of your energy field that resides closest to the gemstone and mineral kingdoms, as well as the sacred plant medicines that grow in Gaia's jungles. The Earth Star is represented by the Mother archetype, the essence of safety and compassion that wants nothing more for you than happiness, safety, and wellness. Let this meditation guide you.

1 / Bring your attention to your feet, and notice the way your feet make easy, intimate contact with the Earth. Curl your toes and then relax them, stretching them out and then curling them in and down to push your energy into the ground. Roll your feet back and push your ankles down toward the ground, curling your toes up and back. Feel the muscles down the backs of your legs tighten as you hold this position. Then relax your feet and let them rest softly on the floor in front of you.

2 / Now imagine that you are walking in a heavily wooded forest. On all sides of you are trees so tall you cannot see their tops. Their trunks are so large you cannot fit your arms around them. Breathe in the forest scent and let the clean, crisp, clear air fill your lungs. Notice how grounded you feel in this moment; it is almost effortless to find safety among the trees.

3 / Return your attention to your feet and imagine the vast strength and power of Mother Earth under them. Think of the centuries, the millennia, for which Gaia has existed, and how much change has taken place on her continents, in her cities, and across her countries. Try to access and pull up as much of that strength and power as you can. Bring up fire and heat from the core of the planet; bring up soil and bedrock and layers of limestone; bring up fistfuls of quartz and tourmaline; pull up fruit and vegetables to nourish and sustain you. Pull up tree roots, branches, and limbs to build a solid foundation for your growth and expansion.

4 / Fill your lungs with the scent of ancient soil, soil that has been buried for hundreds, if not thousands, of years. Once you feel that you can see, hear, and smell Gaia clearly, give thanks for the connection you have made with her. Stay in this space for as long as you feel called to do so.

5 / Say, silently or aloud, "Pachamama, see your children today as they gather strength from your deepest reserves and bless them as they call this energy into present time, into their daily lives, to strengthen, solidify, and support them through change and transformation. Amen, A'ho, So it is." (For more about Pachamama, see page 23.)

6 / With a breath of love and gratitude, release Pachamama's energy from your space by offering words of thanks to her and sending her sweet blessings for her return to the spirit realm.

The Earth Star Chakra is your primary power portal for grounding and stabilizing erratic energies. As the deepest of the lower chakras, it is an important access point for transformative work around releasing, purifying, or transmuting low frequencies. Here you have a sacred opportunity to let go of what is too heavy for you to carry, or what no longer serves your Highest Good. Imagine surrendering these heavy energies and pouring them into the soil under your feet. Take a moment to notice a new lightness of being in your physical body, and sense whether that lightness also extends to your etheric body. You might feel a warmth and tingling in your feet, which are your points of contact with the Earth Star realm. All healers understand the importance of opening and aligning the lower chakras; without a solid and stable foundation in the lower chakras, empaths face psychic burnout. Time spent in the Earth Star realm prevents this, as it re-energizes and nourishes from within.

The Earth Star Chakra is a cosmic buffer: It helps Gaia release cosmic stress from the planet and the immediate environment, distancing you from anything that your physical body cannot integrate or assimilate into healing light. When you allow your Earth Star Chakra to filter out heavy or unwanted energies, or energies that are not relevant or necessary for your training and development in this moment, you take advantage of a valuable resource that is available to everyone, all of the time.

To do this, let go of what is too heavy to carry. Give it back to the Great Mother, whose arms are strong. Next time the cares of the world feel like too much for you, bring your attention to your feet, then to the Earth upon which you stand, then to the layers of rock, soil, stone, and time beneath your feet, then to the bones of the ancestors buried all around you, and send an anchor of light down through the layers. Envision a great anchor made of the brightest white or golden light, and imagine a chain of light extending from your hands to the anchor. Lift the anchor, and let it fall from your hands down to the Earth, watching as it descends beneath the top layers of soil and pushes past, down, through, and beyond where you can see it, bringing its bold illumination to the center of the planet. Let that anchor bury itself firmly on your behalf. Know that nothing you do or say can change the Great Mother's love for, and devotion to, you. Rest in your power and trust that you are always guided and served by a team of guardian Earth Spirits who love, know, and remember you well. This is the medicine of the Earth Star Chakra.

CORRESPONDENCES FOR THE EARTH STAR CHAKRA

goddesses

INANNA, PACHAMAMA

gemstones

BLACK KYANITE, BROOKITE, PETRIFIED WOOD, RED JASPER, SARDONYX, TEKTITE, TIBETAN QUARTZ

tarot card

MAJOR ARCANA: THE HIEROPHANT

rune

OTHALA

essential oils/herbs

BLACK AND PINK PEPPERCORN, CEREMONIAL TOBACCO, FRANKINCENSE RESIN, GALANGAL ROOT, MYRRH RESIN, RED CLOVER, WHITE SAGE

planet

PLUTO

Reflection Questions for
the Earth Star Chakra

Reflective writing is a balm for the soul, and setting the stage for spiritual writing is an intentional process. Light a blue candle for wisdom or a purple candle for spirit guidance. Gather crystals for writing and wisdom, like blue lace agate, azurite, or vanadinite. Then diffuse some essential oils for focus, like geranium or rosemary, and other oils for beauty and peace, like rose de mai or lavender. Brew yourself a beautiful cup of tea in a mug that has special meaning for you: Mugwort tea will soften your consciousness to help you receive spirit messages more easily, while orange tea will bring gentle waves of energy your way and help support a richer attention span.

You might like to choose a special journal or notebook for this process. Choose one that speaks to you or consider decorating one with beautiful stickers or your own art. Choose a lovely piece of vintage ribbon to use as a bookmark. And on the first page, write a brief dedication to your journal—a love note to yourself, reminding you to breathe and relax each time you begin to offer an entry to your journal.

Enjoy the process of setting up your sacred writing space and then let these questions guide you:

1/ Gemstones are the teachers of the Earth Star kingdom. They hold the sacred record of all that transpired on the Earth during the course of their growth, so they have much to impart to us about the history and future of our planet. What wisdom do the crystal and mineral spirits hold for you? If the crystals and minerals could show you where they grew and formed over millennia within Pachamama herself, what stories would they impart? Do you feel a deeper connection to crystals when you think of them as sacred teachers?

2/ What emotions surface for you when you imagine pressing your roots down into Mother Earth? Does the idea of deep grounding inspire or scare you? What potential benefits and risks might come from being more grounded than you are today?

3/ Whereas the Heart Chakra is the heart of the energy system, and the heart of the collective consciousness, the Earth Star Chakra is the heart of the planet. When you place your energy ear closer to our Great Mother, what do you hear? What messages are coming up for you from the depths of the planet? Where is your healing energy and presence needed most now?

When you are ready to close your reflective writing, thank your spirit guides and higher self for attending you while you write, and blow out your candles. Store your gems and other writing tools together in a special place so that you'll have them handy when you want to do more reflective writing in the future.

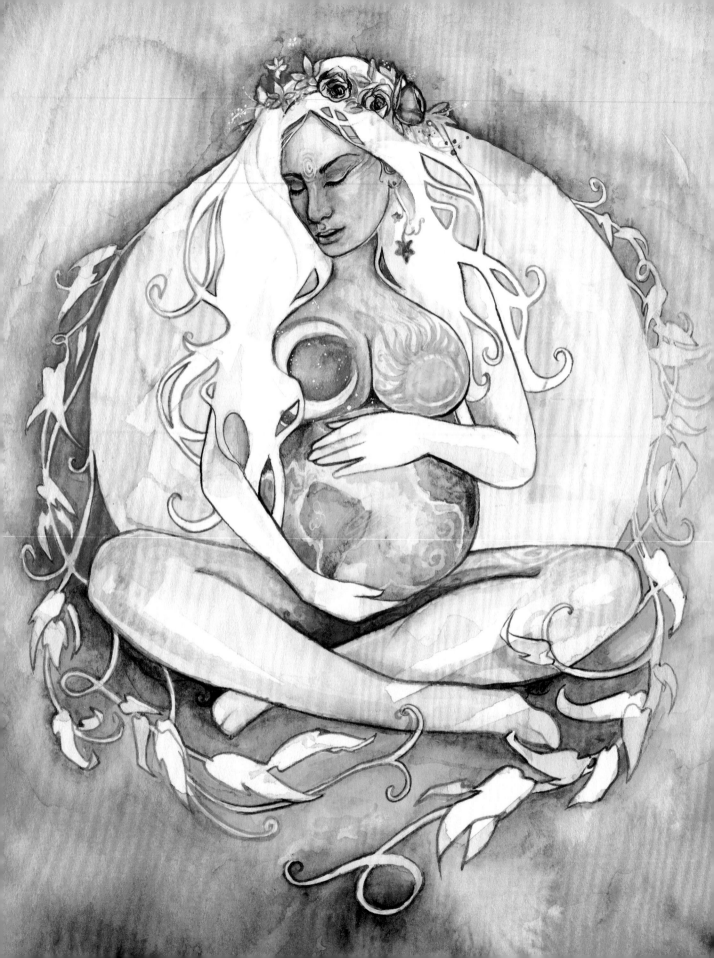

Goddesses of the Earth Star Chakra

Inanna is the ancient Sumerian goddess of creation, and her name means "lady of heaven" in ancient Sumerian Cuneiform. She is also said to be the goddess of sex, beauty, love, wealth, war, and wisdom. Inanna, whose identity became entangled over time with that of the Mesopotamian goddess Ishtar, is the most cited and attributed goddess of any pantheon. She is one of the only goddesses in history whose presence and energy have remained relevant across civilizations. Her ancient and revered status on Earth, and the fact that she governs so many broad and distinct energies, qualifies her as the primary goddess to represent the Earth Star. Inanna is, of all of the goddesses across time, the truest Vasundhara, or daughter of the Earth.

Just as Inanna's identity has transformed over time, shifting from being the oldest goddess on Earth to the most powerful goddess of all things desired by humans—love, sex, wealth, power—you, too, may also have grown and shifted within your own identity over time. How have you encountered and integrated new facets of your power? Call upon Inanna to help you reimagine yourself and safely explore all facets of your identity. (To call upon Inanna, simply say her name. You will draw upon her ancient energy stream and begin to feel her power surround you.) You are, as she was, a brilliant and circumspect creature, capable of shifting and becoming as circumstances require. Let yourself grow, expand, and evolve, trusting that, in doing so, you are safe and protected from below and within. The anchoring magic of the Earth Star Chakra will help you stay steady and centered as you discover the fullness of your magic.

Another powerful goddess archetype with a more modern lineage is **Pachamama**, the Incan goddess of growth, fertility, and natural disasters. In Quechua, the indigenous language of the Andes region, Pachamama translates literally to "Earth mother." Pachamama is the heartbeat and lifeblood of our planet, always fertile and pregnant with new life. She represents the highest evolution of the Divine Feminine and our closest ally in the Mesoamerican spirit world for shamanic journeywork. Pachamama uses her plant and animal allies to create a fortress of strength to support you. Look to her as a grounding force to connect you with Earth energies. Whisper a prayer to her each time you pick a flower or plant a seed. Give thanks to her for strong crops and sacred sustenance. You can even create a small altar to Pachamama in your garden, sprinkling a few seeds to the east as you do, to represent her blessing of new life.

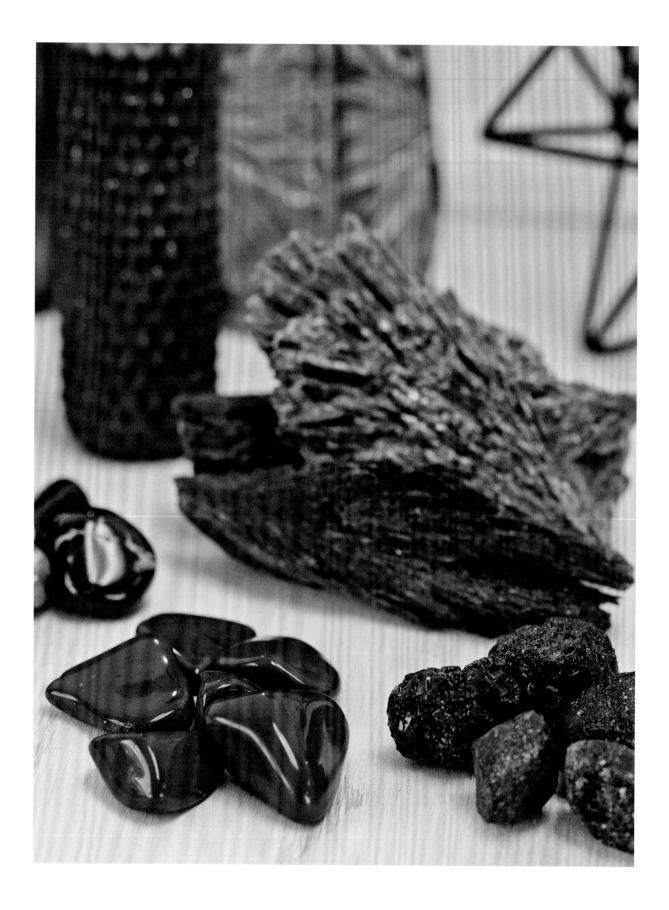

GEMSTONES, ESSENTIAL OILS, AND HERBS OF THE EARTH STAR CHAKRA

Earth Star Chakra Gemstones

BLACK KYANITE clears all energies from all people, places, and things. It serves as the Great Broom, releasing and redirecting energies that are no longer in service of your Highest Good. It is the only gemstone that instantly clears negative energy from all other stones, but does not itself need to be cleared or cleansed. Energy practitioners should keep a piece of black kyanite on their altar to maintain clear energies at all times.

BROOKITE facilitates interdimensional access and, in this way, it allows you to expand your energy field to receive frequencies attuned to other dimensions and realms. These expanded energy frequencies yield access to new layers of wisdom and knowledge and new senses beyond the five traditional ones. Take brookite with you into a shamanic journey or any kind of enhanced or advanced spiritual experience: It will guide you as you expand and integrate a deeper level of awareness.

PETRIFIED WOOD is deoxygenated, fossilized branches and trunks of ancient trees, with their organic elements broken down to reveal layers of quartz under layers of wood. Within the swirls of purple, orange, red, and brown tones, you can find pathways to the magic of center Earth. Ancestors' bones whisper to you from within the core of this sacred gem. Working with this stone—holding it, keeping it with you in your home—will allow it to convey its ancient messages and whispers of inspiration from the distant past.

RED JASPER prepares you for battle, strengthening the blood and internal organs as well as your personal energy reserves and stamina. Native Americans often carried red jasper in times of battle or conflict to ensure resolve and courage.

SARDONYX, the warrior stone of endurance and expanded capacity, reminds you that you are much stronger than you think. Hold this stone in meditation to connect to your inner warrior any time you find yourself in a challenging situation.

TEKTITE is an amazing connection talisman, especially between human souls. It is actually meteoric glass and, as such, contains the grounding of the Earth Star in union with the blessings and ascension energies of the Soul Star. Lovers who must be separated across long distances should hold two pieces of tektite together. Once separated, the two pieces will communicate telepathically with each other, transmitting wisdom and messages to the other.

TIBETAN QUARTZ is the master healer of the Earth Star Chakra. It carries you right back to the arms of the Great Mother, Gaia, so that she can fortify and support you. Working with Tibetan quartz in meditation heals, soothes, and hydrates the physical body.

To work with the Earth Star Chakra gemstones, consider creating an in-ground prayer altar. This is a burial space on land that is sacred to you, in a location where you can safely open a pocket in the Earth about 10 to 12 inches (25 to 30 cm) deep and about 4 to 5 inches (10 to 13 cm) wide.

To create a prayer altar, first decide what you will be praying for. Consider micro and macro prayers; micro prayers are for you, your family, and your home, while macro prayers can be for the entire planet, or even the entire universe. (When you pray, it is wise to hold space both for your needs and the needs of others.) Then gather a few Earth Star Chaka gemstones, essential oils, and herbs (see page 20). Next say a prayer or blessing of gratitude for the Earth and for the fruits she offers you, and for her wisdom and security. Open the Earth in as natural a way as you can, using your hands when possible, to feel your connection to the Earth at this deeper level.

Once you open this sacred pocket of Earth, take one or two of the Earth Star Chakra gemstones in your right hand and blow your breath upon them. Whisper your prayer or request to them as you send them down into Gaia as prayer anchors, holding the energy of the things you desire. For instance, perhaps you are sending down red jasper for strength and courage to help you get through a particularly challenging time or circumstance in your life. Or maybe you are offering Tibetan quartz to your in-ground altar, along with a prayer for healing, to support your own health or the health of someone you love. Take a moment and feel the energies of the stones swirling with the energies of your intentions for the work they will do. Sense the frequency of your intention aligning with the frequencies of the gemstones you have chosen.

You might consider the integration of another layer of energy correspondence by using herbs and essential oils to anoint the stones and the Earth itself. For example, frankincense resin has been used as a prayer offering since Biblical times, and frankincense essential oil is ideal for this task, as are white sage (*Salvia apiana*) leaves. Frankincense grounds the energies of wishes and intentions, helping them take root, and also serves as a sacred offering to Source/God/Creator. White sage leaves are used among Native Americans to clear and purify negative energies and low frequencies from people and places. A single leaf placed into your burial altar, along with a few drops of frankincense or a piece of frankincense resin, adds another dimension of ceremonial magic to this already potent ritual, and helps to intensify the focus of your prayer. Place your stones above the oil and leaf, and then, with your left hand extended palm-down over the hole you have opened, say one final prayer, giving thanks for the blessings that are already on their way to you.

Seal the burial space in as sacred a way as you opened it, filling as much as you can with your bare hands. Feel the gift of Gaia's fertile soil between your fingers as you pray, sing, smile, cry, speak, or whisper your needs—whatever feels right to you. Know that the Daughter of the Earth is listening. She sees you, and she loves you.

Some practitioners recommend revisiting this space one year and one day from the time you bury these offerings; others suggest that a sacred return is not important. Use your intuition to guide you about whether and when you should return to this place, as well as whether and how to care for the space you created. You can leave organic offerings safely within the Earth for a lifetime, so as long as you are comfortable leaving your offerings with Gaia, let them be.

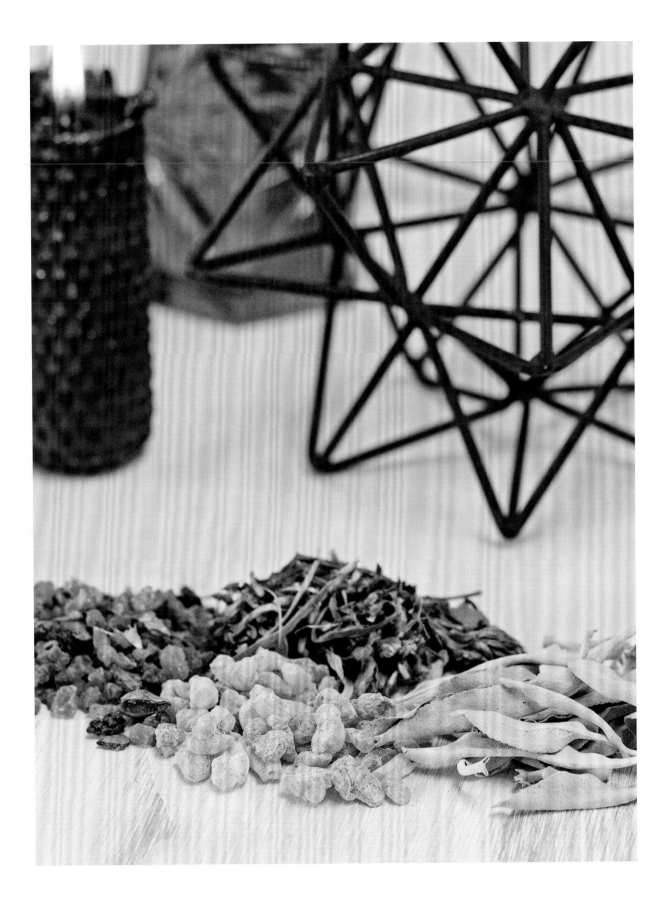

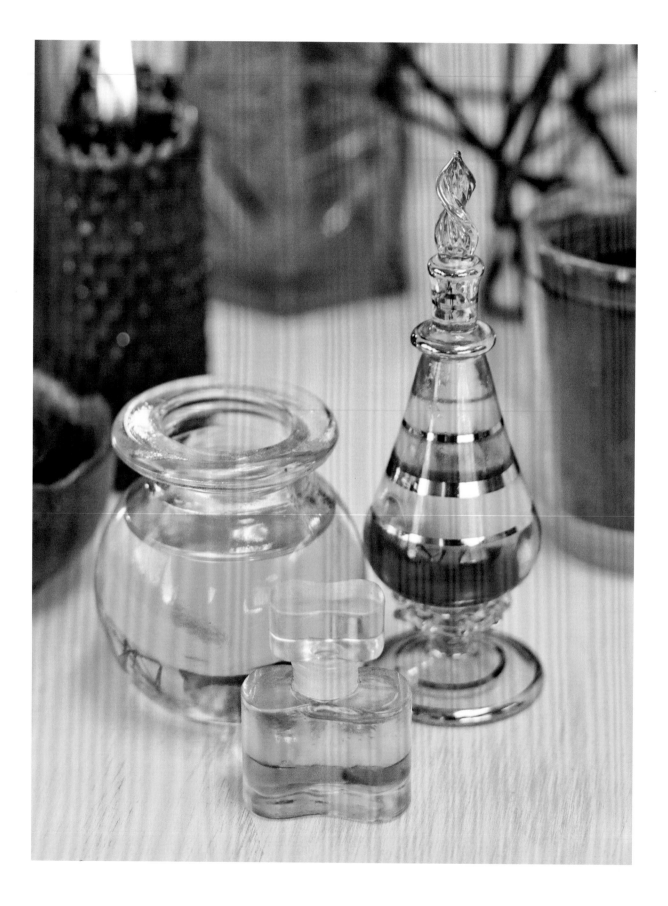

Earth Star Chakra Herbs and Essential Oils

In Native American practice, **Ceremonial Tobacco** is considered a sacred offering to the Great Spirit, and is commonly added to medicine bundles, bags, and pouches, in particular for healing rites and ceremonies. **White Ceremonial Sage** (*Salvia apiana*), when burned, is revered for its power to clear low, negative, or stuck frequencies. Light one end of a ceremonial white sage bundle, blow the flame out, and then place the bundle inside a fireproof dish, fanning the smoke from east to north. Allow the smoke to envelop you and your sacred space, and into it release any energies, sensations, or emotions that are no longer serving you. **Black and Pink Peppercorn**, either in whole, powdered, or essential oil form, bring protection, grounding, and courage. **Red Clover** detoxifies and purifies while **Myrrh Resin** invites angelic energies. **Frankincense Resin** also purifies and is typically used in liturgical practice to prepare for religious ceremonies. Finally, **Galangal Root** facilitates astral projection, as well as contact with spirit guides during divination. It is also very protective of overall physical health, especially the central nervous system.

In Peru, one way to honor the Mother is to create a *despacho*, or organic offering that can be buried within *Tierra Madre*, or Mother Earth, as a way of creating a sacred exchange with our planet. After all, we receive so much from her that it can be rewarding and healing to give something back.

On the following page, learn how to prepare your own *despacho*.

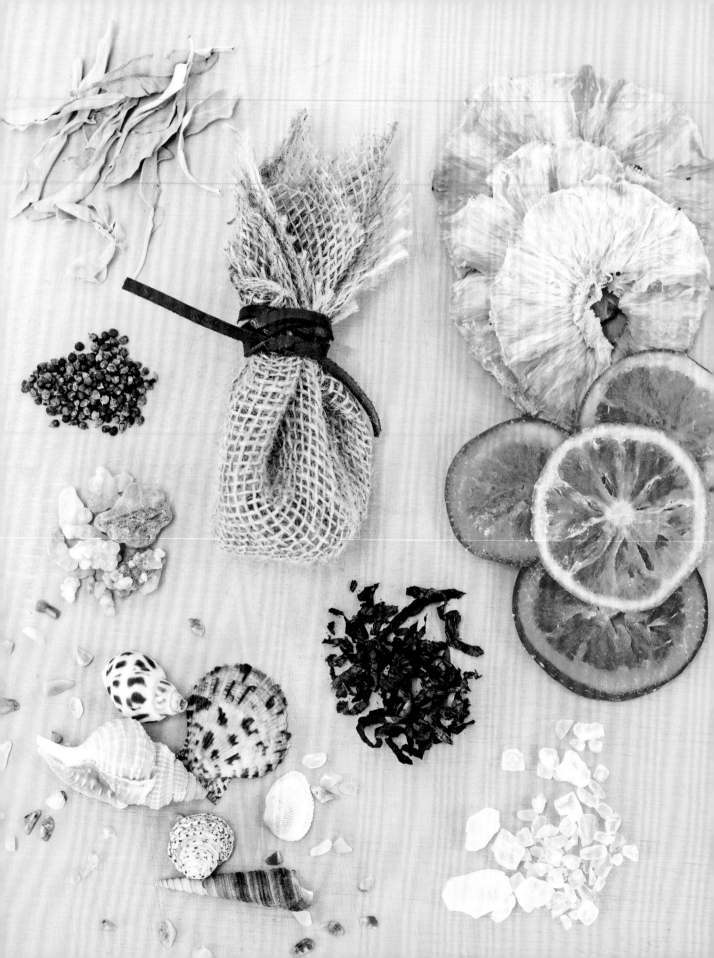

Despacho de la Madre—
An Offering to the Mother

Ingredients

- 1 ounce (28 g) white sage leaves

- Pinch of ceremonial tobacco

- 6 black or pink peppercorns, or a pinch of black pepper

- Frankincense or copal resin

- Brightly colored candies or dried fruits

- Pinch, or one large crystal, of sea salt

- Seashells, gemstones, or other organic materials

- 1 piece (12" x 12" [30 x 30 cm]) canvas or biodegradable fabric

- Twine or thread to tie the package

Make sure that all the items you use are organic and biodegradable, as you will be burying, burning, or floating this *despacho* off to its permanent home—that is, offering it back to Gaia. Include a variety of ingredients, and make sure some are sweet and brightly colored. The Mother enjoys candies and sweets as well as non-edible offerings that bring sweet, loving energies back to Earth.

Place all of the ingredients inside the piece of canvas or fabric, then fold the *despacho* into a square or rectangle. Wrap it three times with your thread or twine, whispering a prayer for our planet each time you do so. Then either bury or burn the *despacho*, or set it out to sea. Release it to the elements and ask that your offering be received by the Mother with love and gratitude—just as it was created. Amen, A'ho, So it is. (While the despacho is meant to honor Gaia, and is not often used for personal intentions, some shamanic groups do create them for group intentions related to Pachamama.)

Tarot Card, Rune, and Planet of the Earth Star Chakra

Major Arcana: The Hierophant

The Hierophant is the keeper of origins and traditions, and is a great teacher of What Was in service of helping you imagine What Is and What Can Be. The Hierophant energies reside in the Earth Star, for this is where your line ascends and descends, and where ancestor bones rest as you integrate their wisdom over time. Here, you locate your cultural origins, and identify with the *terra firma* of Gaia herself.

Call upon The Hierophant to illuminate your view of your ancestors. He is the guardian of the gateway to their bones, your lineage, and shared wisdom. Think of him as the Master Librarian of the Akashic Records, the grand recording of all that has ever happened or will happen in the universe.

If you could access the record of all wisdom across all time, what questions would you ask? What wisdom would you seek from the pages of the Akashic Record? These are profound considerations, so allow yourself a moment here to connect with The Hierophant and to consider what you most need to know at this point in your life and in the development of your soul. Would it help you to know the stories of your oldest ancestors, to become aware of the trials and tribulations they survived in order to find motivation and encouragement? Perhaps you are not sure where your ancestors came from, so your own personal roots are a subject of curiosity for you. In that case, call upon The Hierophant to show you the answers to these questions and help you excavate the ancient ruins of your maternal and paternal lines. Once you know the details of your personal origin story, you will better understand the lessons of this lifetime and how best to navigate them. For example, if some of your living relatives have strong memories of your ancestors and their wisdom, make time to connect with them even if you must travel to do so, for they are the medicine keepers of your line. In meditation, ask your elder spirits and ancestors to share their wisdom with you now in ways you can understand, appreciate, and integrate well into your life. Always give pre-emptive thanks for what gifts might arrive and close your prayer with "Amen, A'ho, So it is."

Rune: Othala

The rune Othala, one of Odin's original twenty-four runes of the Elder Futhark (the oldest form of the runic alphabets), is said to contain the power and energy of all other runes. Othala is also called the blood rune, for it is said to be the chamber of ancestral roots, where the fates of the lines of mother and father are decided. This is the work of the Earth Star chakra because it serves as a filter of parental karmic debt, sparing souls of energies that no longer require purification or re-enactment in the third dimension. You can draw this rune or carve it into wood in order to connect most deeply with its shape and its message. Some people have jewelry with their runes on it, or choose to work with runes via physical tattoo. Whichever way you work with this rune, know that the shape itself carries intense magic and can transfer energy across both space and time.

Planet: Pluto

Even though Pluto isn't technically considered a planet any more, for the purposes of chakras it is. Pluto represents death, transformation, and all that is unseen. The patron planet of Hades, God of the Underworld, in Greek mythology, Pluto illuminates karmic obligations in this lifetime, which are inherited from actions and decisions in lifetimes past. Consider the many ways in which transformation is arising as a theme for you: Are you changing physically, emotionally, or spiritually? All human beings undergo cycles of growth and change; in fact, every seven years, most of the body's cells transform and are reborn. If you are actively seeking support for transformation, look at the house placement and astrological sign in which Pluto sits within your own natal chart. The house will tell you what area of your life is highlighted for transformation in this lifetime, while the sign will help you understand how best to navigate change in your life.

Archetype of the Earth Star Chakra

Archetypes are a concept rooted in Jungian psychology, whereby people enact different faces or aspects of the collective unconscious in their human lives. At the Earth Star, you encounter **The Mother** archetype as you enter Gaia's deepest and innermost chambers. Here, in her tightest embrace, it is possible to experience a powerful awakening. Your capacity for compassion and softness expand, and once they do, you see a way to offer others the love, tenderness, and grace that perhaps you were not offered in your own life. For instance, if you were emotionally impoverished as a child, you may find it difficult to open yourself to affection and compassion in your adult life. If so, the Mother archetype can help you by reminding you of your inherent worth. You are a divine creation worthy of love and sweet affection, of respect and admiration. As you receive this blessing of love from the Mother, you will be less likely to seek out maternal affection in non-maternal places. So much familial and intergenerational healing begins at the Earth Star Chakra.

Mantra of the
Earth Star Chakra

In Sanskrit, the mantra *Om Mani Padme Hum* is perhaps the most sacred of all mantras, since it is said to contain all of the teachings of Buddha within its frequency. It translates literally to "I offer praise to the jewel within the lotus," and it reflects the physical grounding and embodiment of the purest notion of compassion. Repeating this mantra in meditation will connect you with the protective, rooting, and anchoring energies of the Earth Star, and will support you in feeling more connected to Gaia, where healing begins.

Consider what it means to activate all of the Buddha's teachings and blessings with one phrase. Doing so reminds you that, while they are complex, spiritual teachings are also highly interconnected. One of the great lessons to be learned from studying the chakras is the sacred simplicity of energy; it flows seamlessly from one energy center in your body without instruction or direction. Meditate on this concept of simplicity and ease, and think about how you might benefit from deepening your own awareness and compassion. Receive the blessings all around you.

Embodiment Exercise:
Earth Star Chakra Activation

Earth Star Activation is the next step in the process of anchoring your energy deep within the Earth as a means of stabilizing, nourishing, and supporting you. Now, you bring the work back in, back within, toward your center, where you can experience, embody, and integrate this sacred energy frequency in service of mirroring it to the planet. Use this short meditation to guide you.

1/ First, give thanks to the Great Mother, Pachamama, Gaia, Mata, who has given you this life to enjoy and this beautiful planet to care for.

2/ As you give these thanks, close your eyes and let your body relax. Feel every muscle and vertebrae softening, allowing the energies to move through with ease.

3/ Now imagine a beautiful, gleaming, red-black, glowing Merkaba star glowing in front of you, pulsating and shining its red-black light on everything around you. Put your hands out and touch it, and feel the warmth of her Earth pulse as you connect with her frequency. Doesn't it feel like a molten womb, calling you, inviting you home? It reminds you that you are never far from your Great Mother who knows, loves, and appreciates your very being.

4/ Enjoy a moment in her field and then release her back down into the Earth, past the crust and mantle, and down into the core, where she can resume her heartbeat pulse of love and safety. You are never far from her.

Amen, A'ho, So it is. And on we go.

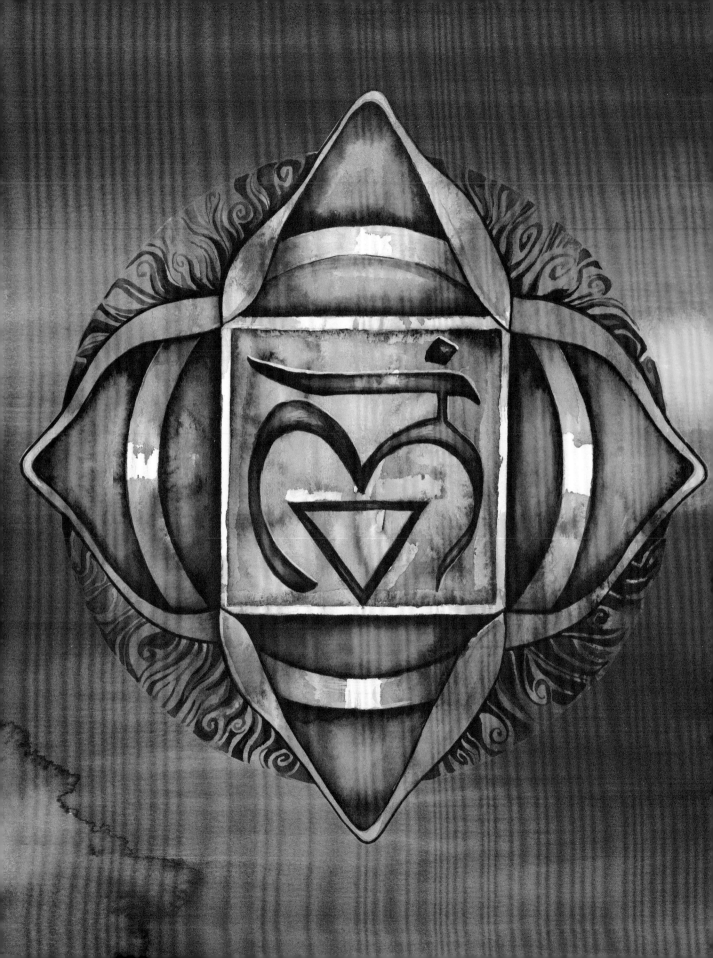

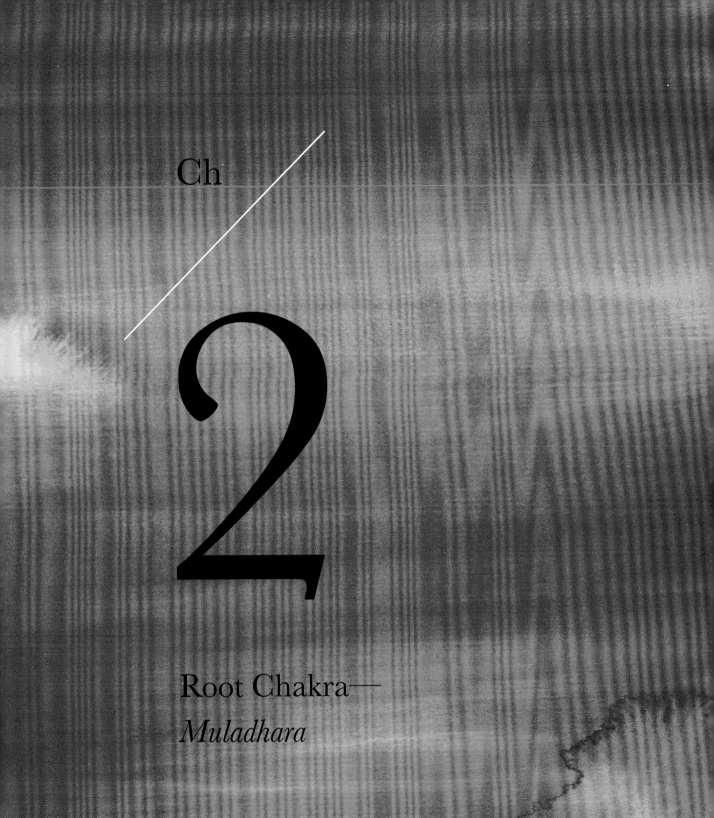

Ch

2

Root Chakra—

Muladhara

The <u>Root Chakra</u> sits at the base of your tailbone and is your center of stability. When it is out of alignment, you feel anxious, nervous, dizzy, or as if you have vertigo. When this chakra is overactive, you feel unable to make progress in your life, on personal or professional levels, and you feel stagnant in your primary relationships. Both extremes feel deeply troubling to you, as if your very life depends on the adjustment.

This is because the Root Chakra is your primary point of balance between the Below and the Above. An unbalanced or unattended Root Chakra can affect every aspect of your life, which is why many energy workers and Reiki practitioners take a bottoms-up approach to chakra work, beginning at the Root (or, even deeper, at the Earth Star) and working upward toward Source channels at the Third Eye, Crown, and Soul Star. When your Root Chakra is active, clear, and functioning well, you are free to move confidently in the world, knowing you are safe, supported, and seen.

In Sanskrit, the name of this chakra, *Muladhara*, means "support" or "root." This is where male sexual energy sits in the physical body (feminine sexual energy sits at the Sacral Chakra). Where the Earth Star Chakra is a portal to the Earthly kingdom of minerals, crystals, and subterranean channels of spirit animals and insects, the Root Chakra is a portal to our relationship with our own physical kingdom—the bodily resources and physical structures that keep us safe in the three-dimensional world we inhabit right now. The masculine energy of the Root Chakra isn't specifically male; it is a protective force field that can bring a deep sense of comfort to anyone, regardless of their sexual orientation or identification. When you learn to connect to the masculine energy stream, you find a steady companion for your journey, one who can ground, stabilize, and direct you toward the best outcome for your work and your life.

In this chapter, you'll learn a great deal about grounding, a concept that's a little more complicated than many people think it is. Lack of grounding remains the number one challenge for empaths and energy workers. Many have yet to learn how to engage the lower and upper chakras all at once, so that while we channel and receive guidance, we can anchor that new wisdom, integrate it, and bring it into embodied form. When you are not grounded, it is difficult to manifest effectively or quickly.

In energy terms, manifestation is the act of bringing thought into form, or bringing your desires into being. The very act of manifestation requires you to engage a deeper density of matter, calling in energies to create new form, which requires a powerful tethering of your energy to the Earth. If you manifest from an ungrounded place, your creations will be temporal and fleeting. Imagine building a house without a solid foundation. You wouldn't even think about doing it, would you? Well, then, neither should you attempt to create or manifest from a place of ungrounded floating in the ethers. I often tell my students to "lift up and root down," a mantra I offer as a reminder that we are equipped with both roots and wings. You are both the Earth and the Spirit. You inhabit both. And so you must create from both.

Embodiment Exercise:
Root Chakra Induction

An induction is designed to help welcome energies, so this exercise is designed to help you inhabit this chakra or energy center and fully experience its gifts. Take a moment and call your energy into present time: Try speaking your full name out loud to call your personal energy in. Bring your attention to this moment. There is nothing to change, fix, move, or shift right now. Your full attention is requested right here, right now. Then let this meditation guide you.

1/ This meditation can be done either standing or lying down. Stretch out your arms, stretch out your legs, and lift your head. Notice how very tree-like your body is: Your arms are beautiful branches, adorned with lovely, leaf-like finger-nails. Next, bring your attention to your legs. They are also strong branches—or, when held together, they are the strong trunk of your tree. Your neck is another branch, lifting your face to the sky so you can receive the beauty of the world, the life force energy of the air you breathe. When you realize how much you *are* nature in every way, you realize that there is no distance between you and The Mother, Pachamama, great and bountiful Gaia.

2/ The Mother figure is one of the most important arche-types, as The Mother is not merely one figure or character in your life; instead, she comes in many forms and as many teachers. Some teach you of the loving, benevolent mother who keeps you safe, nourished, and fed. Others teach you of the dark mother who jeopardizes your well-being through her own selfish actions and desires. The reality of mothering in human form is found somewhere along the spectrum between martyr-dom and abandonment. One model harms us; the other harms the other.

3/ To discern what type of mothering energy is most rele-vant to you right now, sense where in your life or in your energy field you feel neglected. Bring your attention to that place or places. What might help you heal the feelings of neglect you sense? If you do not sense any places of neglect, notice you feel nourished and well looked after. Once you discern whether you are nourished or neglected, you can do a more effective job of balancing Root Chakra energies.

4/ When you balance Earth with Source, when you stand between the Below and the Above, and allow yourself to receive both, integrate both, and be both, you begin to access a deeper layer of conscious awakening. Allow yourself the freedom to be curious about this moment and to notice where you balance the Above and Below within. Ask yourself where you feel most connected to Source energies. How does your connection to each manifest? How do you create balance within your body and externally in your life?

5/ Imagine it now. You are, quite literally, straddling these two worlds even as you read these words. You are the Above and Below in one magnificent form. Allow yourself to feel that power now, that connection. Feel your hips open and imagine the bright beam of white universal light that flows through all beings flowing through and into the soles of your feet, from the core of the Earth, through Gaia and the great Earth Star, up through the Root and remaining chakras, through the Crown to the Soul Star and beyond, out to the farthest galaxies.

6/ Then, see the very top of your head open to the skies, allowing that white beam of universal light energy to return from the farthest reaches of the universe back through the star systems and constellations, down through the Earth's atmosphere and into your Soul Star and Earth Star chakras, through the central column, down through the lower chakras and back … here. Here in the Mother's womb; here in Gaia's uppermost realms; here, where mortals walk, learn, grow, love, laugh, lose, and explore. Here where energy becomes matter.

7/ Here you are. Here it is. Here you can rest, safe, connected, and able to release any energy no longer in your sacred service. Say, silently or aloud, "Guardian Angels, bless us as we integrate the magic and wisdom of the upper and lower realms. Bring us peace as we stand between the worlds and expand our consciousness to reflect universal love and oneness. Amen, A'ho, So it is."

8/ To conclude this induction, take a deep breath. On the exhale, imagine that you are dropping a huge golden anchor down into the Earth below you. As you do, feel the grounding as it strengthens and supports you. Allow yourself to rest here, knowing you are safe, whole, and well. These are the gifts of the Root Chakra. May they serve you well, always.

Reflection Questions for the Root Chakra

Reflective writing allows you a safe and sacred channel for integration of whatever you are learning. Words and writing are so sacred that our ancestors believed every word we spoke or wrote was either a blessing or a curse. So, mind your words, but do use them: The more you write, the more you soften to the process of allowing words to come to you unbidden, and the more likely you are to begin to channel spirit wisdom through your words. In this way, another type of psychic gift becomes available to you.

For now, as you ponder the energy of the Root Chakra, let these questions guide you. You can burn an incense of the Root Chakra herbs, anoint with Root Chakra essential oils, or hold your Root Chakra gemstones while you write, if that feels comfortable for you.

1/ The Root Chakra is the seat of karmic memories—a record of what your ancestors did, thought, and experienced in their lives—and it is the location of the imprints of your ancestors around major issues and energies. When you think about stored memories you experience on a regular basis, what words, phrases, symbols, or ideas come to mind? Keep in mind that stored memories often surface as repeated patterns of behaviors and beliefs. As you begin to question your own internal assumptions, you might uncover some patterns that no longer serve you. Assessing what you take for granted, especially long-held beliefs and entrenched behaviors (like smoking, for example), will help you bring your behaviors and beliefs into alignment with your intentions for health, wellness, prosperity, and peace in your life. Where might you be incubating old or outdated models of working with energies of love, money, work, or happiness that could be limiting you today? If you can access those energies, what messages do they have for you?

2/ How safe do you feel in your life, and why? What or who makes you feel safe and secure? Safety is rooted in the Base or Root Chakra, so it's important to understand your relationship to safety, comfort, and protection.

3/ How do you incorporate nature into your physical routine or sacred spaces? When you want to deepen your connection to Root Chakra energy, it is important to access nature's energy field, either by spending time in nature or by bringing nature indoors in the form of home décor, sacred items you collect on magical hikes through enchanted forests, or gifts that nature leaves for you on your doorstep. For instance, working and decorating with the medicine of peacock feathers (and those of other magical birds) is one way to bring the magic of nature into your life on a daily basis.

The peacock is particularly associated with the Root Chakra. In Greek mythology, Hera, Queen of the Gods and wife to Zeus, had a protector named Argus who had a thousand eyes so that he never lost sight of her. When Argus was killed, Hera placed his thousand eyes on the tail of her favorite bird—the peacock. And so the peacock became Hera's totem creature, protecting her in the same way that Argus had. Think about this story. What protective totems do you treasure in your life, and why? Does peacock medicine resonate with you, and if so, how?

Once your writing is complete, offer a gesture, word, sound, or other offering of gratitude to your spirit guides and higher self for attending you while you write. Keep your gems and other writing tools together in a special place so they are handy when you want to do more reflective writing in the future.

CORRESPONDENCES FOR THE ROOT CHAKRA

goddesses

PELE, KALI

gemstones

BLACK TOURMALINE, JET, ONYX, RED AVENTURINE, RED JASPER

tarot card

MAJOR ARCANA: THE WORLD

rune

ALGIZ

essential oils/herbs

ALLSPICE, ANGELICA, BURDOCK, CAYENNE, CEDARWOOD, CLOVE, DANDELION, NUTMEG, PAPRIKA, ROSEMARY

planet

SATURN

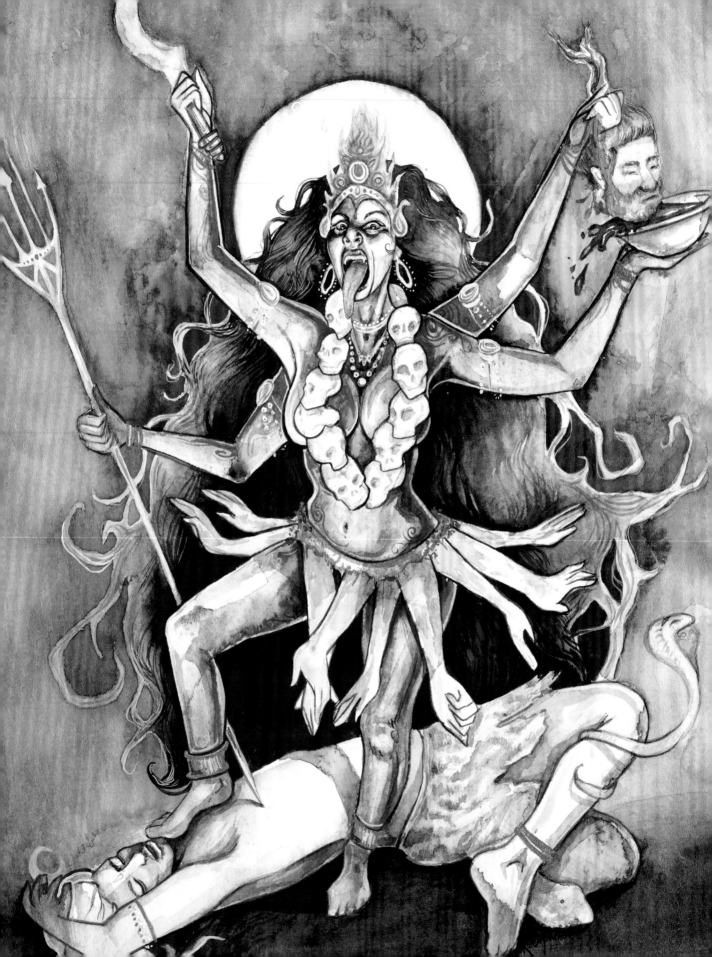

Goddesses of the Root Chakra

Pele and **Kali** are the two primary goddesses of the Root Chakra, but they are also goddesses who work with the element of fire in order to manifest, to transform, and to create. Pele hails from the Hawaiian pantheon—she is keeper of the fiery cauldron of lava from which the Hawaiian island chain was born—while Kali is the Hindu goddess of death and transformation.

To work with these goddesses, you must begin by entering their ancient domain—the Earth—with reverence. This means that you are called to walk carefully upon the Earth, taking only what you need and leaving this planet more beautiful than you found it. One way to pay homage to the great goddesses is to begin seeing yourself as a divine creature, elevating the way you speak to and about yourself. When you treat yourself with deep respect, it becomes second nature to treat others and the Earth accordingly. Once you demonstrate your reverence in this way, both goddesses will open themselves to you, allowing you to warm yourself by Pele's fire and meet Kali's transformational gaze.

When a deity makes itself known to you, you may begin seeing symbols related to her more frequently, or you might sense her energy in meditation. When you seek goddesses such as Pele and Kali, you begin to see echoes of them in even the most mundane details of life. You can turn to either of these deities in times of fear and insecurity, such as illness, personal or political crises, or periods of transformation and change, for both are capable of assuaging your mortal concerns.

Both goddesses use destruction as a tool of creation, facilitating new beginnings through the conscious release of what no longer serves you. Be cautious as you work with these deities, however, if your intentions are unclear. Approach them with reverence and awareness of their powerful lineages. These are warrior goddesses who protect by virtue of their own powerful energy fields, where the cycles of birth, life, and death turn sometimes violently upon themselves. Because death is a natural extension of life, these goddesses invite our connection with all cycles of life and seek to attune you to the fullness of creation. Once you release fear of their potency, you will find them to be helpful allies who summon in you the same fearless fire that attracted you to them in the first place. Commit to standing fully in your power as you engage them and theirs.

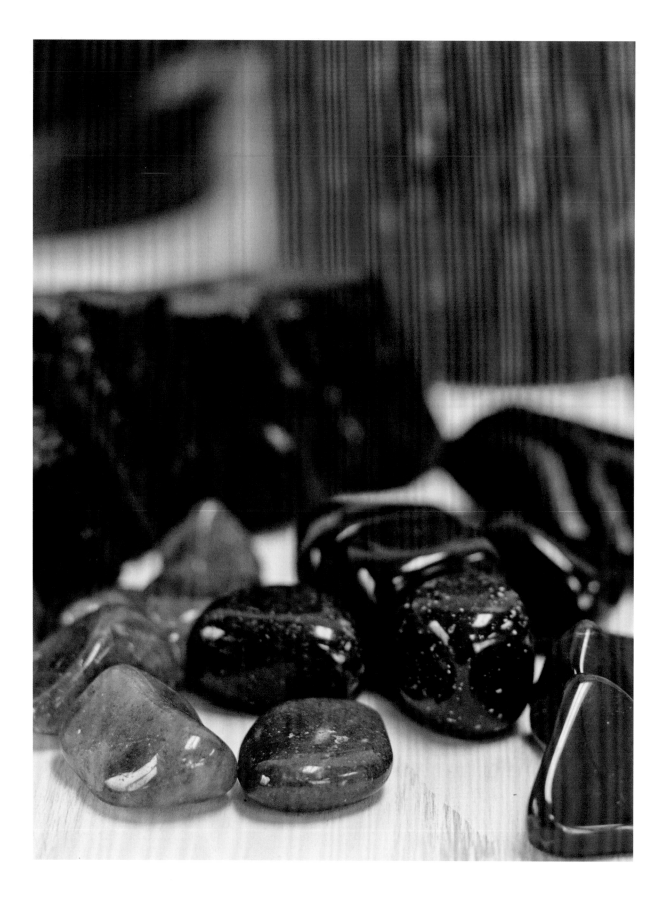

GEMSTONES, ESSENTIAL OILS, AND HERBS OF THE ROOT CHAKRA

Root Chakra Gemstones

BLACK TOURMALINE guards its keeper and her property with the utmost care and devotion. It is the most protective stone in the mineral kingdom. Place four pieces at the four corners of your home or property to protect your home and land, and keep a piece in your car to prevent theft.

JET is a product of wood that is decayed and deoxygenated under high pressure. Although it is light in weight, jet packs a heavy punch when it comes to protection, removing curses or hexes, and filtering dark magic that stems from previous ages or lifetimes. Our ancestors believed that carrying a piece of jet would help protect them from disease, including the Plague.

ONYX helps empaths as a working tool by absorbing and transmuting low vibrations within people or places. It is believed to make the bearer physically strong and invincible, and to attract good luck and a strong harvest.

RED AVENTURINE purifies and detoxifies energy frequencies to help clear stored trauma, promoting a deeper connection to Source energy. It helps facilitate strong circulation in the body, releasing stored toxins and improving blood flow.

RED JASPER is a stone of strength in battle and reminds the bearer of her personal strength and fortitude to resist challenges. Native Americans believed that red jasper strengthened warriors who were heading into battle. Its red color represented the blood they would not have to shed due to the stone's protective properties.

To work with the Root Chakra gemstones, consider making a Safe Surroundings Medicine Bundle to help ground and stabilize you. To begin, find a piece of fabric that has a special meaning for you—perhaps a piece of an old T-shirt you loved, or a piece of your child's clothing, or an abandoned but much-loved blanket. Ideally, this piece of fabric should be about 4 square inches (26 cm²) so that it can hold two to three tumbled stones as well as any herbs you may wish to add. Also, gather twine, silk ribbon, or a beautiful thread to tie the bundle closed.

When crafting a medicine bundle, always let your intuition guide you about what to include. When you do, you might reach for items such as photographs, seashells, gemstones, pieces of jewelry, or other things that surprise you. Trust your intuition as you do this. If you are called to include something, it is because that item is meant to work with you right now; it has something to teach or show you that is worthwhile. You might not know why at the moment, but down the road, in hindsight, it will likely make more sense than it does now.

Once you have gathered your medicine bundle items, place them in the center of your fabric square. Be sure that all of the ingredients are safely captured within the bundle. Be mindful as you add each piece, whispering prayers of intention for peace and protection as you go. Once all the items are safely inside, pick up each of the four corners of the fabric square. Bring them to the center, and then fold the bundle in on itself to make a rectangle or square "envelope." Wrap the bundle with the twine, ribbon, or thread three times before tying a bow. (In magic, the number three represents the triple goddess, the three primary phases of the moon, the three faces of God—Father, Son, Holy Spirit—and much more.)

When you have tied the bow, blow your breath of life across the bundle and give thanks for its medicine. Carry it with you or keep it on your altar. Some people keep their medicine bundles with them for years, if not decades, while others bury their bundles, burn them, or release them into the ocean. Listen to your spirit guides for counsel about how best to work with this sacred tool, and trust your intuition. It is most traditional to bury a medicine bundle once it is complete, as long as all of the ingredients are biodegradable. May it serve you and protect you well.

"

...DANDELION IS CONNECTED TO THE UNDERWORLD AND IS SAID TO FACILITATE EASY COMMUNICATION WITH THE DEAD.

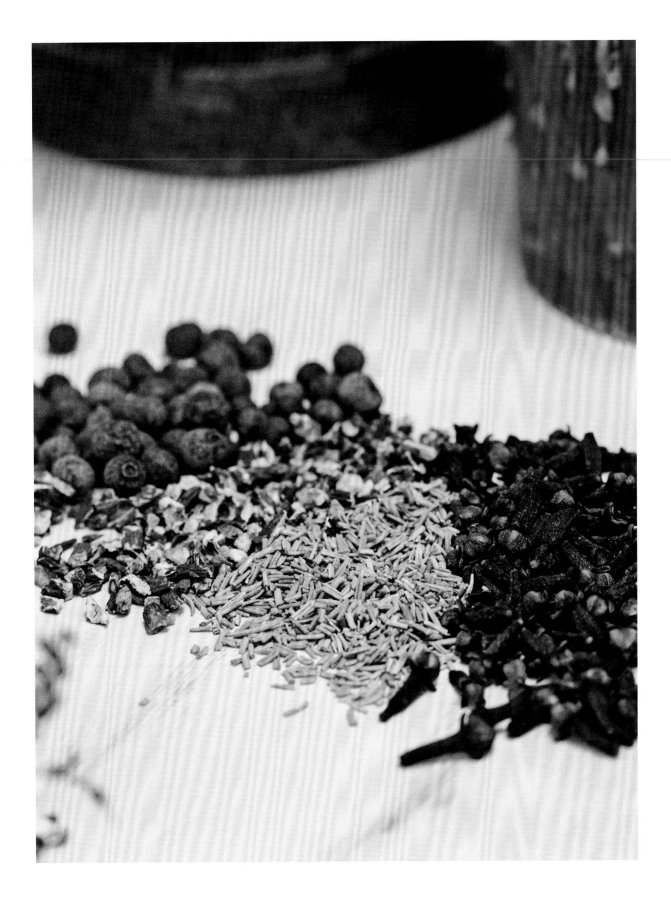

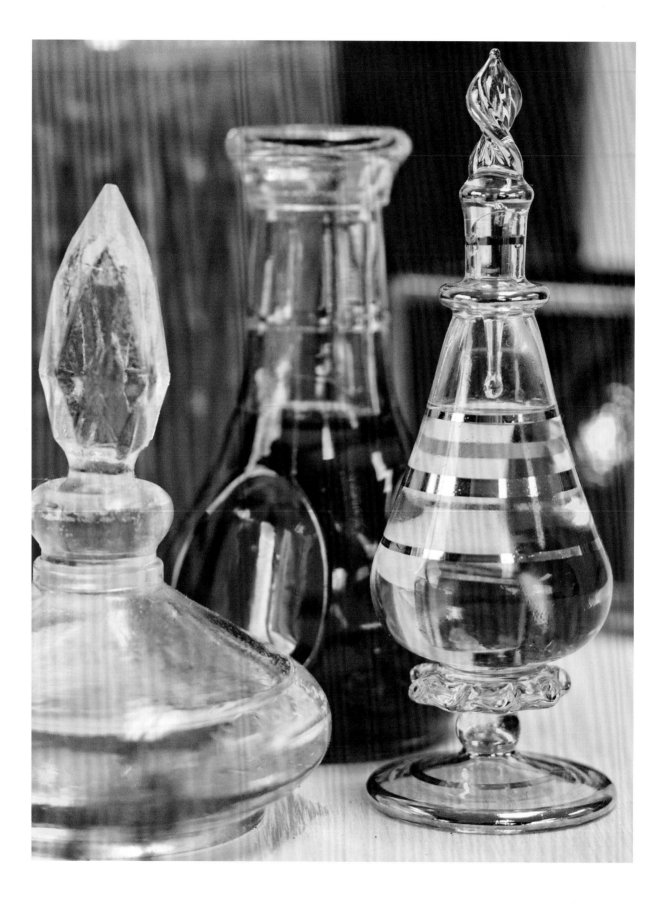

Root Chakra Herbs and Essential Oils

Burdock brings prosperity and strength, but also cleanses the aura of negative thoughts and vibrations, and is especially helpful with negative inner monologues. **Clove** brings protection and attracts what you seek; it also helps you connect to memories of love or safety from childhood. **Dandelion** is connected to the Underworld and is said to facilitate easy communication with the dead, while **rosemary** helps clear stuck energies and entities from spaces. **Paprika** is energetically grounding and helpful to empaths who need to avoid holding onto the energy of their clients. **Cayenne** has similar properties to paprika, but is also helpful for cleansing and purification rituals. (Cayenne can also boost the spice in your love life—no pun intended!) **Allspice** draws money to the bearer and ensures good fortune. **Nutmeg** ensures loyalty and luck, while **cedarwood** grounds and strengthens the physical body. Finally, **angelica** protects both people and property, helping filter out the influence of negative entities—especially in trauma, where a life ended tragically or unexpectedly.

One way to work with herbs and resins without consuming or burning them is to arrange them in a beautiful, sacred, repeating pattern in your garden or on your altar. Herbal mandalas like these can be left in place for weeks at a time before being taken apart and then ritually burned or scattered to release the energies once the work is complete.

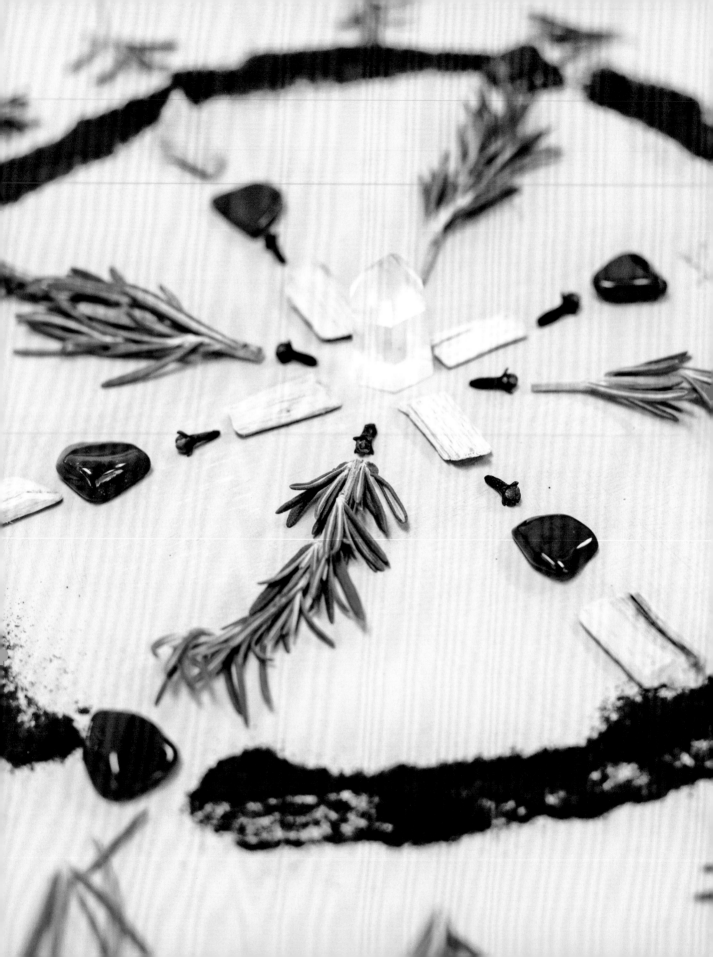

Sacred Protection Herb and Resin Mandala

Ingredients

- 8 whole cloves
- 8 sprigs of rosemary, fresh or dried
- 8 cedarwood chips
- Cayenne, paprika, or allspice powder for sprinkling
- Quartz points and Root Chakra gemstones, if desired

Before creating your mandala, think about the appropriate location for your design. Will it be a temporary space, or would you prefer to leave the mandala in place permanently? This will help you decide whether to work indoors or outdoors. Next, think about what kind of protection you seek based on the elements, and let that decision guide the directional placement. Do you seek the protection of ancestors? If so, create a north-facing mandala. Do you seek the protection of clear sight and freedom of thought, or a new beginning? If so, create an east-facing mandala. Do you seek the protection of strength in battle? If so, create a south-facing mandala. Do you seek emotional protection? If so, create a west-facing mandala.

Then, lay out all of the herbs and resins in front of you, and ask for guidance about how to arrange them. Avoid overthinking this: Let Spirit work through your hands instead. Try laying out four pieces of each herb, spice, and resin first, one in each direction. Then divide the quarters in quarters again with the remaining pieces. Place the rosemary sprigs at the cross-quarters between the spices and resins. Sprinkle the loose spice and herb powders around the mandala, creating patterns as you go. (When creating a mandala, you always want to place objects with intention to create repeating patterns.) Once your mandala is pleasing to your eye, you are finished. Give thanks for the inspiration and magic it represents, as well as the protection it will bring to you and your space. Amen, A'ho, So it is.

Tarot Card, Rune, and
Planet of the Root Chakra

Major Arcana: The World

In the Tarot, The World card is said to denote the cycles of time and nature, and the impact of both time and nature on the human experience. In many ways, The World represents the union of Earth and Source—the mingling of the metaphysical with the mundane—that characterizes the Root Chakra. The main theme of The World card is integration, for it represents the amalgam of tools and resources necessary to build an empire. All knowledge of the past, present, and future meet in The World card, and can be harnessed for your use. The main question asked by The World card is, "What do you desire most?"

If you could access all that you desire, and if you were able to fully integrate the spiritual with the mundane in your life, what would that cosmic integration look like? So many people are unable to manifest what they seek simply because they do not believe their desires are attainable. You might feel that way, too. But just for a moment, allow The World card to open your mind and your heart so that they can hold space for what seems impossible. Your belief is fuel for your dreams. Such is the medicine of The World.

Rune: Algiz

Algiz is one of Odin's original 24 runes of the Elder Futhark (the oldest form of the runic alphabets). It represents the overarching protection of the universe that is available to all humans at any time. By uttering the word or drawing the symbol of this powerful rune, you too can harness its protective energies, for it forms a protective shield over you, keeping you safe from the storms of life. Whether your fears are physical, emotional, or spiritual in nature, you can turn to the energy of Algiz to calm and comfort you. Let its energy pour over you like a virtual shield of energy.

Algiz carries the vibration of the Valkyries from the Norse tradition. They are the female warrior spirits who carry out Odin's divine will on the battlefield, deciding who will die in battle and who will survive. The Valkyries are strong figures of protection who often saved soldiers' lives on the battlefields when their mortal journeys were not yet complete. In this way, the Algiz rune reminds you to trust in the energy of the Valkyries, for they will protect you in times of danger and can save your spirit on the battlefields of life. During an especially challenging period in a relationship or at work, for example, you can connect to the Valkyries and ask that they deliver you safely to the other side of whatever obstacle you face. They can carry you through and help you connect to energies of bravery, courage, and strength.

Planet: Saturn

Saturn is the father of the solar system, the great teacher of what must be and the bearer of life lessons. At the Root Chakra, Saturn affirms the importance of stable rhythms and cadence in life and the role of structure in your personal and spiritual development. Order and moderation in all things is the law of Saturn. Saturn tightens the noose on us energetically, forcing development rather than letting it unfold on its own terms. If you fall out of line or do not complete the tasks of life, Saturn reminds you of the gaps you overlooked and then requires you to complete what is undone, closing energy loops. Knowing this, you can anticipate some of the Root Chakra challenges and work to overcome any natural inclination to leave tasks incomplete. By noting where Saturn falls in your personal natal astrological chart, including the house Saturn sits in as well as the sign governing Saturn for you personally, you can better understand how parental energies are likely to manifest in your own life.

Archetypes of the Root Chakra

Here, at the Root, you are invited to discover **The Guardian Angel** and **The Soldier**, two different but aligned faces of protection that manifest in people, places, or the experiences that you choose (or that choose you). The Guardian Angel archetype provides protection through wisdom and deep access to hidden understandings. For many, the Archangels—and in particular, Archangel Michael—are also archetypes of the Root Chakra.

The Soldier, on the other hand, is able to keep you physically safe by forcibly protecting your spaces through acts of aggression. (When working with protection archetypes, it is important to recognize that one's face is non-violent while the other's is violent. Without judgment, we recognize that some transgressions in life require action for protection and some require diplomacy.) Both the Guardian Angel and the Soldier offer shelter from the worries and challenges of mortal life. Their method of entry and *modus operandi* are different, but their intention is the same: your protection and safety. As you encounter the Root Chakra archetypes, let yourself soften into the role of child and surrender your major worries and concerns to them. Where can you learn to trust more deeply that all is well, and that you are supported, held, and protected? What parts of your life or health would improve if you made fewer of your decisions based on fear?

Call upon these energies when you are feeling tired, discouraged, or weak. Imagine them as strong allies to you who can take from you the anxieties, hesitations, and insecurities that keep you from feeling strong and stable in your life today.

Mantra of the
Root Chakra

In Sanskrit, the mantra *Aad Guray Namay* means "I bow to the primal wisdom [of Source]," and is considered to be a mantra of the White Light of Divine Protection. It is thought that by honoring the divine wisdom of the planet, you become able to walk in that wisdom—indeed, to walk through it and inhabit it, thus lessening personal human suffering and erasing human fears. When you feel scared and alone, simply uttering this mantra will bring you closer to God (regardless of how you conceptualize the Force that created you, and by whatever name you summon it). The recitation of this mantra is also said to attract new teachers to you, in addition to new sources of wisdom and protection.

Consider what it means to send out a universal request for new teachers or new pathways to learning. Doing so creates space in your life for new energies and new people to arrive who can offer you new insights and ways of deepening your spiritual practice. What would you like to learn, how, and from whom? Meditate on the many ways you might benefit from deepening your own practice and expanding your toolkit. Give thanks for the wisdom already on its way to you.

Embodiment Exercise:
Root Chakra Activation

Root Chakra activation is one way of accessing a deeper level of connection to the Earth to help stabilize your energy centers and strengthen your energy reserves. Then you can begin the sacred task of integrating the wisdom of this protective energy center, this pulsing center of swirling red light that is like a beacon of safety and wellness. Use this short meditation to guide you.

1 / First, know that when you rest in the space of the Root Chakra, you are home. There is no need to seek peace outside yourself. Give thanks to the protection goddesses and your spirit guides who guard you daily. Give thanks also to Archangel Michael who comes to guide you toward the light of love and protection in your life. Say, thank you, thank you, thank you.

2 / Just as you would crawl into your mother's lap as a child at the end of the day, or after a stressful event, so you can now crawl into the Root Chakra. Imagine yourself curling deeply into a fetal embrace, holding yourself as you are held within the planet, within the solar system, and by ancestors whose bones lie below you and whose spirits fly above you.

3 / Let yourself curl up and in, and know it is safe to rest here and now. It is safe to believe that dreams can come true and circumstances can change in your favor, quickly, and without force or toil. It is safe to allow the river of your life to flow without feeling the need to force it here or there? The river is not waiting on your command and does not require your permission to flow. If you feel uncomfortable in any way, speak softly to yourself the way you would speak to a small child who was afraid. Remind yourself that all is well, here and now.

4 / Here at the Root, it is not only safe to let go, it is also the law. You must surrender. Choose surrender. Do not wait for surrender to choose you. The easier path is the path of allowance. As you think about allowance, notice any areas of discomfort or resistance you encounter. Acknowledge the resistance, then consciously release it and let it go. Keep talking to your child self. She is safe to allow. She is safe to trust. She is safe to be. Breathe in this allowance: It is the Great Mother's gift to you. She wants you to enjoy the one life you've been given—this life. Treasure it, guard it, appreciate it. Use it for the good of all.

Amen, A'ho, So it is. And on we go.

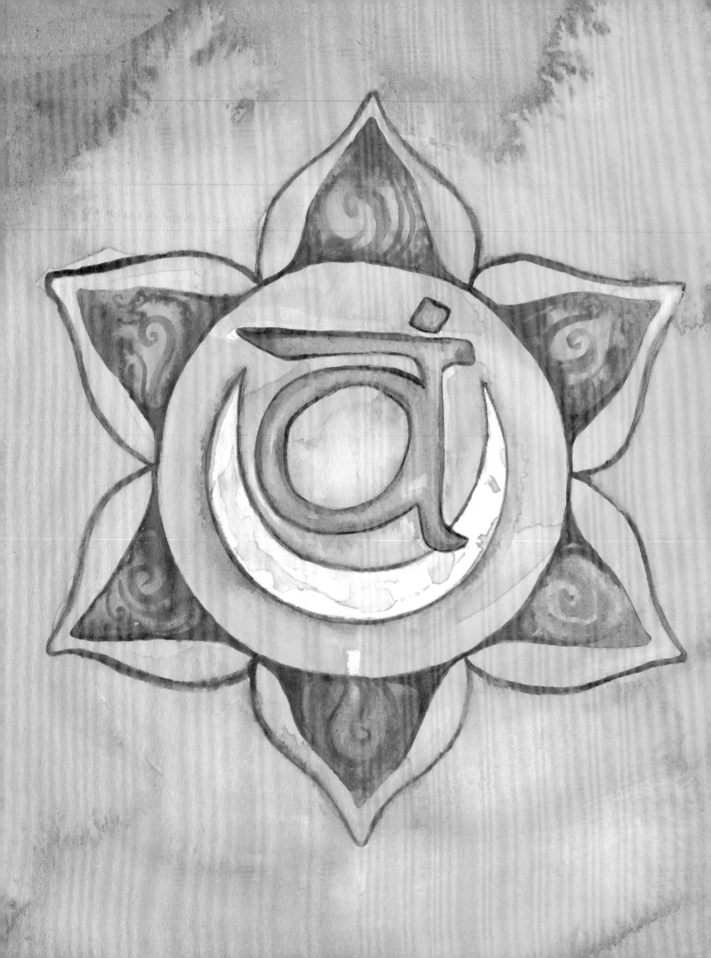

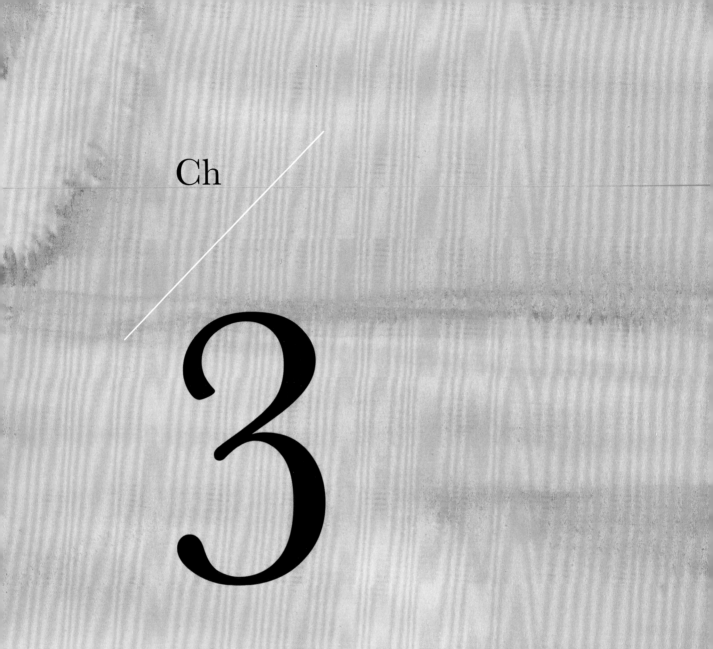

Ch

3

Sacral Chakra—
Svadisthana

The Sacral Chakra sits between the reproductive organs, in the center of your lower abdomen, and represents the life force of creative potential. Here is the domain of creation and procreation, the well of potential for what will be. When the Sacral Chakra is blocked, or isn't spinning with ease, your sense of creative potential is blocked. This might manifest in an apparent lack of inspiration for a creative project; an inability to pursue your art, or a loss of interest in it; or physical infertility.

In many cases, Sacral Chakra blocks last for years, if not decades, and in Western cultures are often thought to be associated with age. Many people think it is natural to lose inspiration, sexual desire or passion, and the ability to conceive a child with age. While there are natural physical limitations to childbearing, you can (and should!) receive inspiration and desire sexual intimacy well into the later years of life. After all, the best years of life are often the later years, when earned wisdom shapes experience and helps prevent the mistakes of youth. So, too, should the later years of life be full of laughter, intimacy, and creative exploration.

At the Sacral Chakra, it is possible to heal trauma from sexual abuse in the past or present, as well as medical procedures like hysterectomies, Caesarian sections, and abortion. Healing sexual trauma as a means of overcoming infertility or boosting creativity may seem strange at first, but everything is related in energy work, bound by region of the body and center of energy. Anything you bring into being in this life—whether it is a child, a new idea or invention, a project, some kind of service to others, or leadership in any capacity—is governed by the Sacral Chakra.

For many women, blockage in the Sacral Chakra leads to the closing-off of sexual intimacy in relationships and can have far-reaching consequences, including depression and loss of hope as well as separation and divorce, in dire cases. If this sounds familiar, know that help is on the way! This chapter offers tips and strategies for opening and healing this important energy center. Your vitality—and, thus, your happiness—depends on it. You are meant to live a full, sexy, vibrant life.

Embodiment Exercise:
Sacral Chakra Induction

This Sacral Chakra induction is designed to help introduce you to the energies of this chakra, which governs all creative and procreative endeavors. If you are ready to explore the art and the passion of your life, this is your chance. Use this short meditation to guide you.

1/ Become mindfully aware of your thoughts now, and bring them into this moment. Notice the objects around you, the Earth beneath you, and take a moment to look around your life and recognize how many of the people, things, and structures in your life exist because *you* made them. Yes, you! To connect here at the Sacral Chakra, it is important for you to view yourself as a sacred, creative vessel of inspiration, a veritable fountain of passion and desire that overflows into all aspects of your life. You might imagine your desire and your passion as rivers of water or flowing lava from an ancient volcano. Visualize your deepest essence pouring out of you like water or liquid fire, nourishing or melting everything in its path. You are tapping into a river of your own power. Feel it bring you to life, one cell at a time.

2/ Some believe that sexual energy is only necessary in a relationship with a partner, but in fact sexual energy is the currency of the entire universe. Every being, every vibrational creature understands and responds to sexual frequencies. This means that seduction is about honoring the value of what you have to offer, and sharing it with others from a place of deeply shared desire for connection. That connection can be emotional or physical, or it can simply be a neutral vibration without attachment. When you see yourself as the Seductress, as the one who enchants and seduces, how does that feel? Let the energy of the Seductress drape itself around you like a gorgeous velvet shawl. Feel its soft warmth around you and then consider how you can bring that luxurious sensuality into your life.

3/ Ask yourself which experiences in your life today bring you pleasure. Make a mental list of those activities or experiences, noting the ones you have engaged in within the last twelve months. Then, commit to bringing more of these experiences into your life. If you are in a relationship, consider involving your partner in this inventory. It can be very exciting to bring shared passions and desires to life!

4/ Once you have connected with the energies of the Seductress and identified the desires you wish to access and fulfill, give thanks for the blessings these desires will bring to your life. So begins the cycle of abundance and prosperity, rooted in faith, trust, and sweet surrender.

By consciously reconnecting with your ability to desire and be desired, you will feel empowered, and empowerment fuels health, self-esteem, and, by extension, happiness. Thus, doing the work of the Sacral Chakra—while sometimes painful and difficult, especially if childhood trauma is triggered—is still very much a worthwhile venture. When you align and clear the Sacral Chakra, your entire life receives an infusion of passion and creative courage. Get ready to feel alive and inspired! Nothing is more important, because no one is more important than you when it comes to your soul's development. It's time to put you first.

CORRESPONDENCES FOR THE SACRAL CHAKRA

goddesses

BASTET, ISHTAR, RATI

gemstones

CARNELIAN, GOLDSTONE, IMPERIAL TOPAZ, ORANGE CALCITE, PEACH MOONSTONE, SHIVA LINGAM, SUNSTONE, TANGERINE QUARTZ

tarot card

MAJOR ARCANA: THE EMPRESS

runes

URUZ, KENAZ

essential oils/herbs

BLOOD ORANGE, CINNAMON CASSIA, FENNEL, GINGER, TANGERINE, VANILLA, YLANG YLANG

planets

JUPITER, MERCURY

Reflection Questions for the Sacral Chakra

As you begin to ponder the questions in this section, ask your spirit guides to support you in channeling wisdom from your higher self in order to receive a download that can guide your practice. To do so, close your eyes and imagine yourself in the center of a circle. Then, imagine that the circle is formed of spirit beings, each of whom has a divine connection to you—as a guardian, an ancestor, or an ascended master teacher. Ask them to support you as you explore your passion and your creativity and to offer sacred inspiration to guide you. (If you are unsure what your passions might be, ask your spirit guides to show you through signs and symbols.)

Gather a few tools to accompany you as you journal and reflect. Reach for carnelian and blue lace agate, which will raise a powerful creative vibration. Or, brew a cup of Sacral Chakra tea by infusing damiana, ginger, and fennel in hot water for 5 minutes, inhaling the spicy aroma before you sip and enjoy the warming herbs. When you are ready, let these questions guide you:

1 / How has your sexual desire and physical passion changed in the past year? How are you relating on a physical level to your partner, or to yourself if you are not currently in a relationship?

2 / When you consider the archetype of the Seductress or Enchantress, notice the emotions that emerge for you. Remember that in ancient times, the concept of sacred sexuality was alive and well: Sex was considered to be one way to raise a powerful energetic frequency that could then be channeled in different directions to manifest will. To which areas of your life could you direct the flow of your sexual energy in order to manifest what you desire? Where do you need to "loosen up" and let go in your life, feeling less concerned about what others think and becoming more mindful of your own desires?

3 / What does intimacy mean to you? What intimacy do you enjoy in your life right now, and in what parts of your life do you desire deeper intimacy with others? If you could instantly manifest your desires for intimacy right here and right now, what would that look like?

When you are ready to close your reflective writing, thank your spirit guides and higher self for attending you while you write, and blow out your candles. Store any gems you've used and other writing tools together in a special place so that you'll have them handy when you want to do more reflective writing in the future.

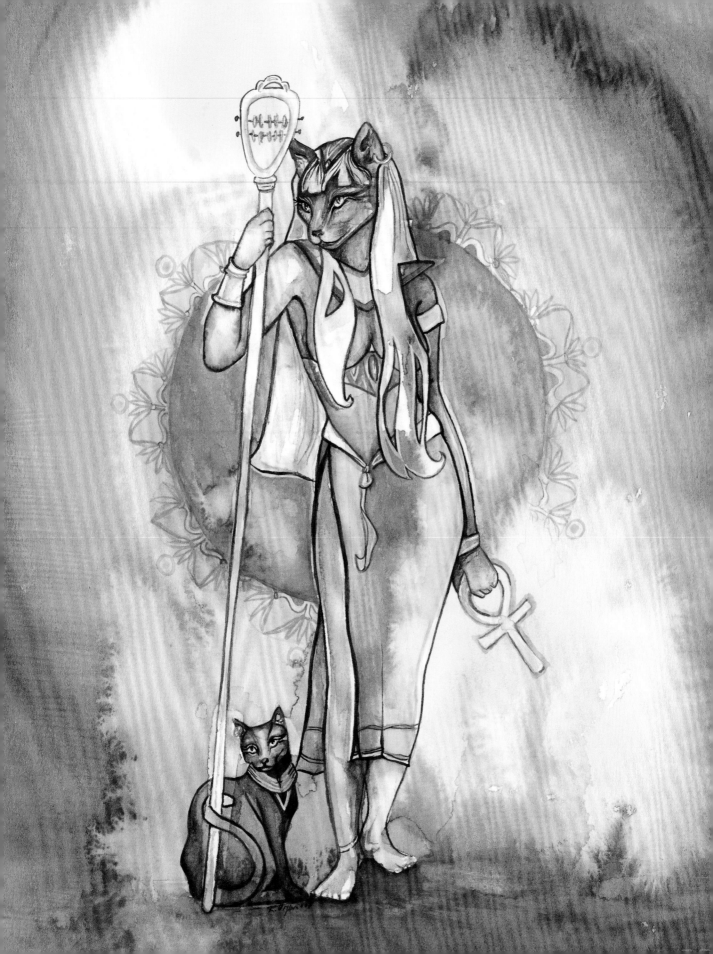

Goddesses of the
Sacral Chakra

Bastet, **Ishtar**, and **Rati** come forward as the goddesses of
the Sacral Chakra, and have much to teach about the sensual
power of passion and desire. Rati is the Hindu goddess of
love, lust, and physical desire, as well as sexual intercourse and
the physical union of Divine Masculine and Divine Feminine.
Ishtar was the famed Mesopotamian goddess of desire, and
the tales of her lusty adventures continue to inspire women
today to connect with their innermost sensual selves. Within all
women lies a (sometimes dormant) goddess of sex and desire;
the key is to liberate and summon her, welcoming her energy
into all aspects of your life and honoring it as sacred. Bastet,
daughter of sun god Ra in the Egyptian pantheon, is the
supreme goddess of pleasure. A feline goddess who is depicted
with a cat's head, she governed sensuality and pleasure of
every kind. Simply setting the intention to work with these
goddesses and to bring more of their subtle, seductive, and
feline qualities into being will help you to access their energies
in your own daily life. You can also call upon them by name,
followed by the words, "Be with me now."

> ...A FELINE GODDESS WHO IS DEPICTED
> WITH A CAT'S HEAD, [BASTET] GOVERNED
> SENSUALITY AND PLEASURE OF EVERY KIND.

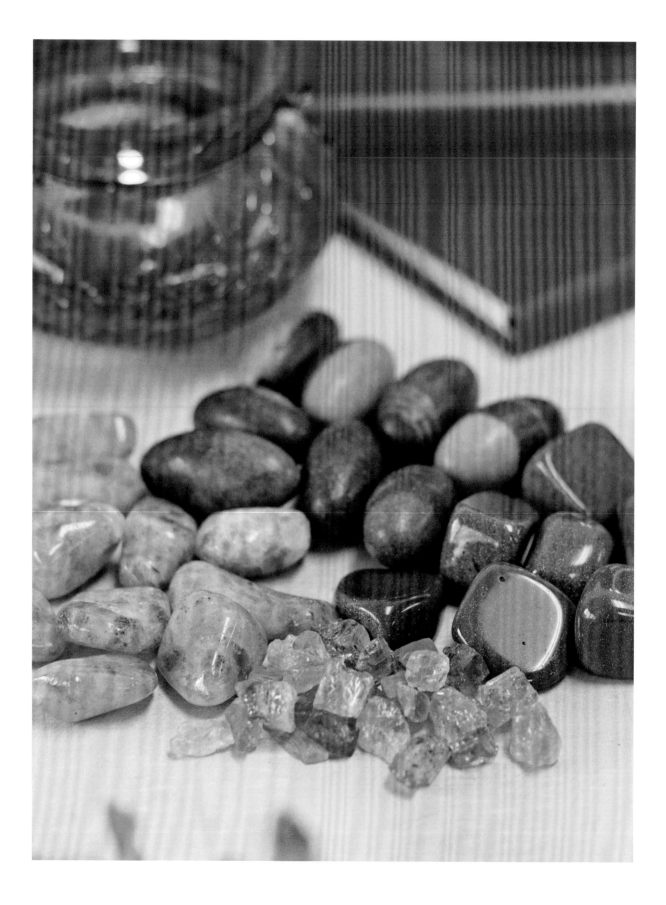

GEMSTONES, ESSENTIAL OILS, AND HERBS OF THE SACRAL CHAKRA

Sacral Chakra Gemstones

CARNELIAN is the gemstone version of caffeine, giving you a turbo boost of energy to help you stimulate creativity and complete even the most arduous of tasks. If you need to move more confidently in the world, use carnelian as your secret empowerment weapon.

GOLDSTONE contains natural copper and thus supports healthy circulation. Goldstone conducts energy beautifully, and so it can help you feel more balanced, aligned, and empowered. Hold it during intercourse to improve blood flow and strengthen the intensity of orgasms.

IMPERIAL TOPAZ, one of the rarest of all topaz colors, is a deep orange talisman of strength and power. Its fiery orange glow is linked to its reputation as an aphrodisiac.

ORANGE CALCITE is said to help with erectile dysfunction and sexual performance issues. Men report that orange calcite facilitates sexual stamina and endurance, while women report that it helps counter the effects of menopause on sex drive. **SHIVA LINGAM** represents the sacred integration of Divine Masculine and Divine Feminine energies.

PEACH MOONSTONE harnesses the creative powers of the moon phases. It is thought to represent the waxing gibbous moon phase that is most often aligned to manifestation.

SUNSTONE is the leadership stone for politicians, teachers, and managers of all kinds. It activates the fire within, helping you connect to untapped potential and enthusiasm.

TANGERINE QUARTZ boosts sex drive and brings sexy thoughts of lusty connection to the bearer. It is believed to be an aphrodisiac that can support male sexual performance and improve sexual endurance.

Consider working with your Sacral Chakra gemstones at sunset, as Sacral Chakra energies are most heightened in the early evening hours. Lie down comfortably, removing shoes or other items that feel restrictive to you, and then place your Sacral Chakra gemstones across your lower abdomen, either in a circle or in a line—whatever feels most comfortable and aligned with your intuition. Next, stretch your arms out to your sides and imagine a bright orange ray of light beaming down to you from the Sun. Warm and potent like the Sun itself, it casts its orange ray of heavenly creative light across the stones you have placed, charging and infusing them with universal wisdom about passion and connection. Give thanks for this burst of light wisdom and commit to embodying it every day as you walk your path. And so it is.

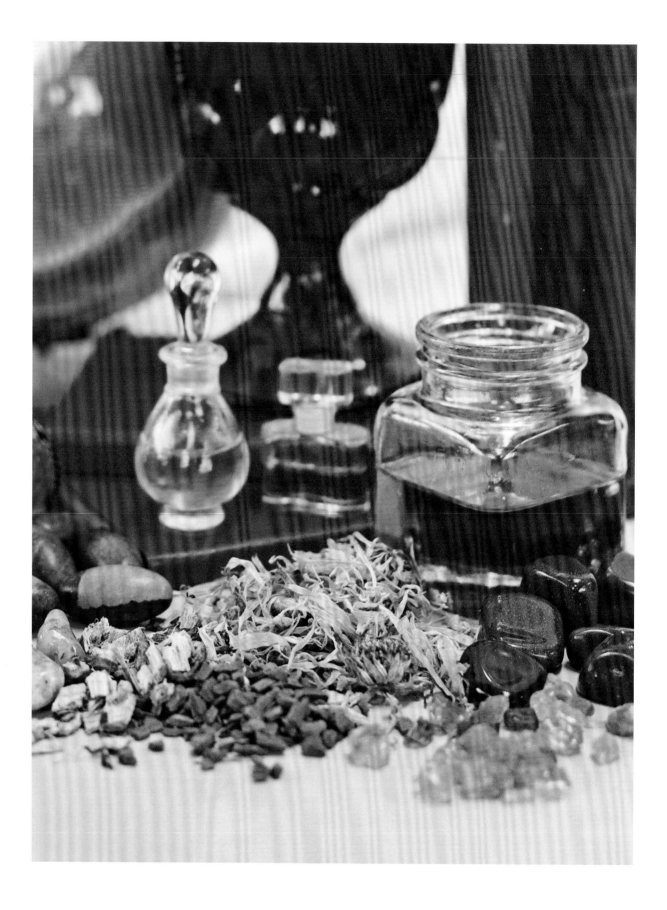

Sacral Chakra Herbs and Essential Oils

Ginger helps create a stronger flow of chi through the reproductive organs to stimulate sexual passion and interest. **Cinnamon cassia** boosts metabolism and purifies the system, while **blood orange** brings welcome energies of joy, prosperity, and power. **Tangerine** reconnects you with the Inner Child, helping you feel more innately playful, happy, and carefree. **Ylang ylang** is nature's most potent aphrodisiac after Damiana and offers an added benefit of enhancing intuition. **Vanilla** is the queen of the orchid family and brings you a sense of sweet benevolence, activating energies of peaceful leadership and selfless service. Last but not least, **fennel** eases digestive troubles while enhancing memory.

Many of these herbs and fruits can be used in teas. Citrus tea is a perfect wake-me-up, while ginger tea helps soothe sore tummies and activates creative energies. Diffuse vanilla resin or ylang ylang essential oil in your home to invite sweet spirits and help create a calming, enjoyable environment for guests. (That said, the combo of vanilla and ylang ylang is extremely seductive, so use it wisely!)

During the holidays, try making the recipe on page 71 to activate the energies of the Sacral Chakra fruits, herbs, and spices while adding some Yuletide magic to your home environment.

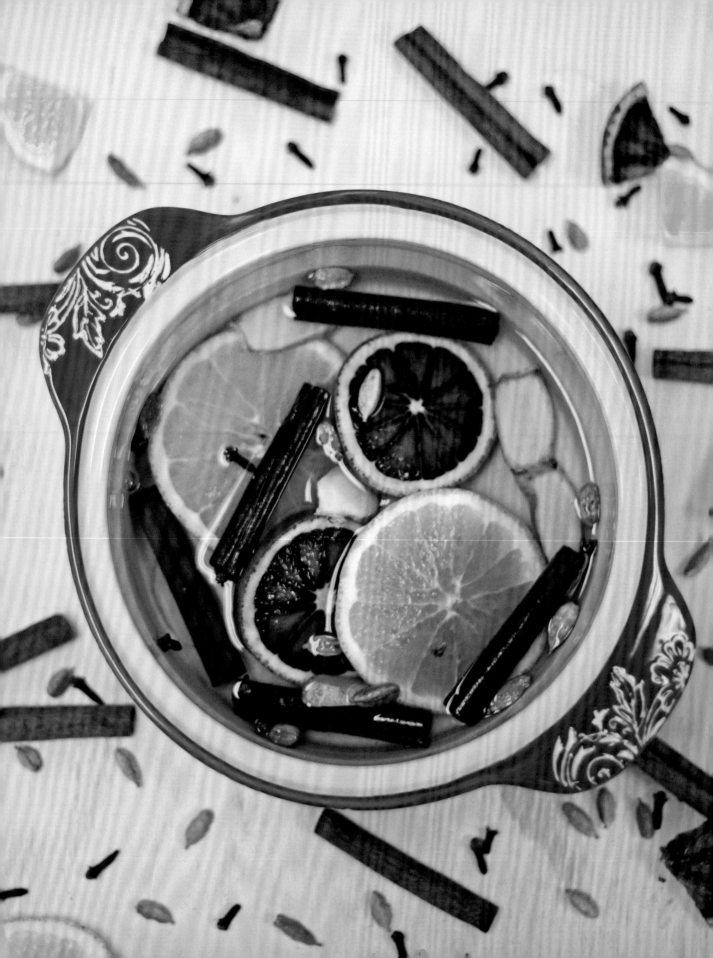

Yuletide Simmering Herbal Blend for Sensuality, Inspiration, and Creativity

Ingredients

- 4 blood oranges and/or orange slices
- Fresh ginger, sliced
- 10 whole cloves
- 5 cinnamon sticks
- 10 cardamom pods

Bring a few quarts of water to a gentle boil on your stove, then reduce the heat to a simmer and add all the ingredients to the water. Your home will be filled with the most enchanting yuletide scent, but you and your guests will also enjoy energies of prosperity, happiness, comfort, joy, and health. Let the blend simmer for as long as you like, adding more water if necessary. You can also simmer these herbs in apple cider or red wine, then strain out the fruit slices and herbs before sipping. Amen, A'ho, So it is.

Tarot Card, Rune, and Planet
of the Sacral Chakra

Major Arcana: The Empress

The Empress is the Mother of the Major Arcana, pregnant with life and possibility. Seated in her velvet robe of beauty and aesthetic magic, she represents luxury and manifestation. She is also the only figure in the Major Arcana who is carrying a child; in this way, she comes to represent both motherhood as well as the capacity to birth other energies, such as new projects. She is the embodiment of creative potential. Connect with The Empress to express more of your maternal or creative power, as well as your divine beauty.

To connect with The Empress, imagine yourself as a fertile, pregnant being, full of life and possibility. What would it look like for you to be full of a new idea or new project, incubating a concept or gestating a new piece of art? What are you meant to deliver or give birth to in this lifetime? The Empress wants to know. Sit for a moment and speak to her of your desires. She will fuel them, inspire them, and help you carry them safely until it is time to bring them fully into the world in material form.

Runes: Uruz and Kenaz

Uruz and Kenaz are the runes of personal success, power, and deep understanding. The mantra of the Sacral Chakra is "I create," and it is here that your deepest understanding of your purpose in this lifetime becomes manifest. Uruz ensures that whatever you create will be met and received with success, and Kenaz helps you to cull the lessons from what you create, so that you continue to learn as you manifest new life and new projects. When you are in the initial stages of a new project or new idea, call upon Uruz and Kenaz to support you and inspire you from within. Both of these runes facilitate success with any new beginning.

Planets: Jupiter and Mercury

Jupiter is the planet of manifestation and creation, so it makes sense that it's one of the planets of the Sacral Chakra. Seeing Mercury, the planet of communication, here may be a surprise to you, but Sacral Chakra work requires you to access your voice and communicate your desires in order to gather the resources you need. If you can dream it, and if you can communicate it, you can create it!

Jupiter is the planet representing evolution in your own time. Where Saturn demands timely development and evolution, Jupiter holds a gentler expectation of your growth: Here you are free to grow on a timeline that serves you. Mercury's forward and retrograde motions bring you opportunities to practice communication and then to reflect on where you might be able to improve your communication skills.

With both planets, learning is not only allowed but encouraged, and reflection becomes a natural part of the learning process. After all, the Sacral Chakra sits on the threshold of the lower and central chakras, the gateway to a higher level of conscious awareness.

Archetype of the Sacral Chakra

The Temptress and **The Saint** emerge as the archetypes of Sacral Chakra energies. The Temptress is the part of you that feels her deepest desires in a visceral way and longs to share that physical passion with a partner who can meet her halfway. She also serves to strengthen your confidence and mirror your beauty to you. The Temptress is not just a seductress in the realm of sex or physical expressions of desire; she also represents the broader temptation to all kinds of pleasures, worldly and otherworldly.

The Saint is a figure on the other side of the desire spectrum who hides her desires, sacrificing them to the needs and desires of the Greater Good. Sometimes the Saint emerges out of need or circumstance, when life demands that your needs come second (or third, or ninth) to those of others around you. However, the Saint is a reminder of the dangers of not honoring your own needs as sacred, for the Saint cannot manifest or create without channeling her passion. The Temptress, then, emerges to inspire you while the Saint in some ways is a reminder never to let go of your needs, even if you must prioritize others at certain times in your life. You matter, too. You stand between Saint and Temptress, giver and receiver of pleasure.

Mantra of the
Sacral Chakra

Samba Sadashiva is a Sanskrit mantra written in homage to the Lord Shiva in the Hindu tradition. He is the divine partner to Shakti, with whom he represents the whole of Creation. Shiva represents what must be erased or destroyed in order to create. Think of the things, people, places, or experiences that have had to melt away from, or transform in, your life for you to ascend to new levels of spiritual development. Think of what you have had to release with grace in order to welcome what is new. Even though it is always difficult to suffer a loss of any kind, especially when what you lose is dear to you in some way, remember to move as quickly as possible to a place of gratitude, for without loss you would not know the power of receiving. When you let go of what no longer serves you, you create new space for growth, permitting the Universe to fill with all the things you desire now. You have already let go of so much that has weighed you down; give yourself a sweet hug and reflect on the processes that have led you to this moment. Then, let yourself feel the building excitement of what lies ahead in your life. You have only begun to tap your creative potential.

Embodiment Exercise:
Sacral Chakra Activation

Sacral Chakra activation helps you initiate a series of energy events to prompt a stronger flow of energy to and from this particular chakra. If your passion center has been dormant, now is the time to awaken and receive the wisdom of the Sacral Chakra. Use this meditation to guide you.

1/ First, know that so much is ahead of you and so much stored energy waits to take form through you: with your hands, through your heart, in your mind, through your womb. As you consider the many ways in which you express your given creativity, dream for a moment about creative outlets you have not yet explored. Where in nature are you finding sacred inspiration? Perhaps it is the changing color of Gaia's leaves this season, the swath of colors at this evening's sunset, or the stark simplicity of a smooth, gray sea on a rainy day that will inspire you to consider new ways of connecting to the beauty around you.

2/ Move back into the present moment. Allow yourself the gift of feeling your physical desires. Summon your inner Temptress and bring her seductive, mysterious, irresistible fire to your awareness. Then imagine summoning the energy of the fire element for courage, stamina, and strength. Feel the power of the ancient Divine Feminine rise within you: It is the essence of queens, rulers, priestesses, and wise women of all kinds from all places across all time. They seek connection with you, and they seek to create through you. You become an open channel for their cosmic wisdom. In this way, you not only channel the Divine Feminine, you become the Divine Feminine. Your womb gestates art, beauty, and life.

3/ Now allow yourself a moment to enjoy what you have seen and experienced. You are so divinely beautiful and vibrating with possibility. Give thanks to your spirit guides, guardian angels, and ancestors who are also celebrating your passion and potential. Know that you are the product of many centuries and generations of love. Amen, A'ho, So it is.

May you always know the depths of your own beauty, your own passion, and your own creativity.

Amen, A'ho, So it is. And on we go.

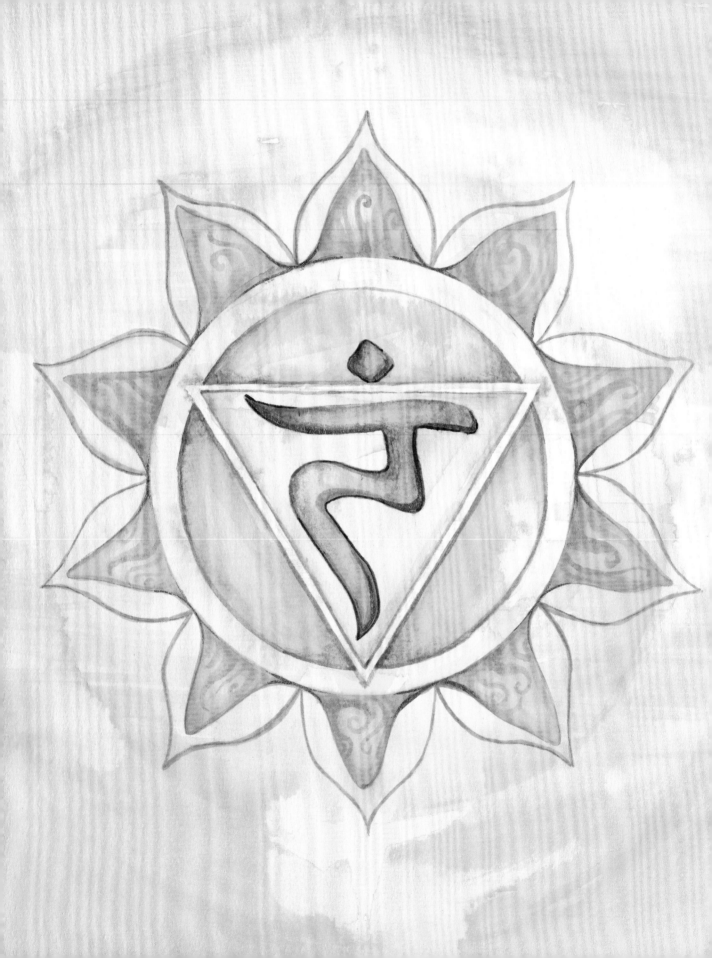

4

Solar Plexus Chakra—

Manipura

The <u>Solar Plexus Chakra</u> sits two finger-widths above your belly button, in what is called the Power House of the energy field—your energy center of power and confidence. When this chakra is well-balanced and aligned with the rest of the chakras, you feel empowered, confident, and capable. It is the key to manifesting what you create at the Sacral Chakra. Think of the Solar Plexus Chakra as the key that unlocks the door you built in chapter 3. In this chapter, you will step through that door and reap the rewards of your work.

There is much fulfillment to be had at the Solar Plexus Chakra. But there are cautionary tales to tell as well. An imbalanced Solar Plexus Chakra can lead you to feel either powerless or omnipotent, both of which are states of confusion and potential danger. As the saying goes, all things in moderation. In order to use your power wisely in life, for the Greatest Good of All Beings, you must temper power with humility. Humility is the medicine the Solar Plexus chakra offers.

Embodiment Exercise:
Solar Plexus Chakra Induction

The Solar Plexus induction is designed to welcome you to your deepest sense of personal power. For some of you, it may have been decades since you honored or recognized yourself as a powerful being. That's okay! As you bring your attention to this moment and prepare to engage the energies of the Solar Plexus Chakra and your own personal power, consider how the Sun is, in many ways, a mirror of the Solar Plexus Chakra. Solar energy emits a beautiful, warm, comforting, golden light that is also the light of inspiration, manifestation, and offers you a deep sense of strength and power. Use this short meditation to guide you.

1/ To open your connection to the Solar Plexus Chakra, imagine sitting in the middle of a tropical beach on a sunny day. Feel the air swirling around you, warming you from within and without. Notice a gentle breeze moving through, just enough to keep you comfortable. Feel the sand under you, surrounding and comforting you.

2/ Now imagine the sun above you, sitting in center sky, beaming down upon you. Each ray is a source of power for you, a place where you can expand and become. Receive those rays: Let them flow down upon you from above, on the top of your head, your shoulders, your arms, and your hands. Close your eyes and be nourished by this connection with the sun. All forces of light are now with you in this moment. They are here to strengthen you and remind you of your own power and competence. You have the skills and wisdom you need to move forward powerfully in your life, make good choices and decisions, and manifest what you seek.

3/ By consciously connecting with your own personal power at the Solar Plexus Chakra, you also empower those around you to explore their potency as well. In this way, as each person finds her power in this life, so the entire collective becomes empowered to rise. Sense how your own inner sense of royalty, your own inner sense of sovereignty, becomes active now. You are so ready for the next chapter of your life to unfold. Feel that excitement, and step boldly through the door before you. This is your time. Everything has been guiding you here.

4/ When you feel fully prepared to walk through this door of possibility, invite any ancestors or spirit guides who wish to accompany you. Feel their presence as they surround you, and trust that they will offer any wisdom you need to progress safely to the next level of your development. Close your induction with the universal blessing: Amen, A'ho, So it is."

Reflection Questions for the Solar Plexus Chakra

Power, in our society and in many of our mental models, is typically associated with the Divine Masculine and is thought to be a more natural energy stream for men to access than women. However, the original civilizations of our planet were matriarchies, in which women found power in formal positions of authority and leadership. Though we live in Western society, many of us remember on a soul level what another, more fluid, form of leadership looks and feels like. Are you ready to tap into your well of personal power? If so, brew a cup of herbal tea with Solar Plexus herbs to support you, such as calendula, lemon, anise, and turmeric. Work with pyrite and citrine to activate the Solar Plexus Chakra and summon solar energies for deep alignment with power, purpose, and a positive perspective. Then, ask your spirit guides to be present with you as you consider and respond to the following questions:

1/ Where do you exercise your personal power in your life? When you think about your own power, what images come to mind?

2/ How would you describe yourself as a leader, and as what sort of leader would the people in your life describe you? Do you lead more effectively at home or professionally?

3/ What does leadership mean to you? Can you identify positive role models—in any context—who inspire you to carry your leadership in a different way, perhaps in a way that is more deeply aligned with who you are and what you value?

When you are ready to close your reflective writing, thank your spirit guides and higher self for attending you while you write, and blow out your candles. Store any gems you've used and writing tools together in a special place so that you'll have them handy when you want to do more reflective writing in the future.

CORRESPONDENCES FOR THE SOLAR PLEXUS CHAKRA

goddesses

MA'AT, SEKHMET

gemstones

AMBER, CITRINE, COPAL, GOLDEN CALCITE, GOLDEN HEALER QUARTZ, ORPIMENT, PYRITE, TIGER'S EYE, YELLOW AVENTURINE, YELLOW FLUORITE, YELLOW JADE

tarot card

MAJOR ARCANA: THE EMPEROR

rune

THURISAZ

essential oils/herbs

ANISE, CELERY, CINNAMON, CUMIN, GRAPEFRUIT, HELICHRYSUM, JUNIPER, LEMON, LILY OF THE VALLEY, MARSHMALLOW, MELISSA, MINT, NEROLI, TEA TREE, TURMERIC

planet

SUN

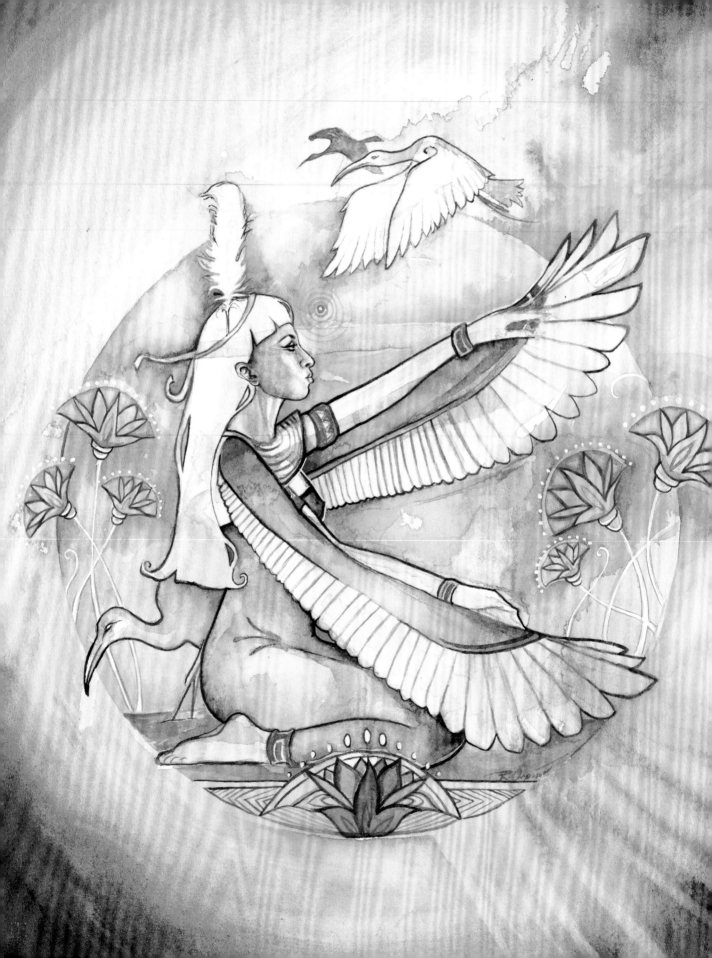

Goddesses of the Solar Plexus Chakra

There are many goddesses of power, and therefore of the Solar Plexus Chakra, and each face of power they represent speaks differently. You will identify with some more easily, or more profoundly, based on your life experiences. **Sekhmet** is the golden sun goddess of the Egyptian pantheon who rises in the East, the direction of dawn and the Solar Plexus. **Ma'at** is her counterpart in the Egyptian pantheon, patron goddess of justice and fair outcomes. Diana and Athena come forward from the Greek pantheon, goddesses of the hunt and wisdom, respectively.

These two goddesses harness the elements in service of your empowerment; their focus is your perfect balance of elements and energies. When you need more energy, they can summon fire to give you a burst of southern directional energy for focus, will, and strength. When you need inspiration, they can blow the winds of the east in your direction, helping you to breathe more deeply into the moment and find your center. Call upon these goddesses when you feel overwhelmed and incapable of completing the tasks before you. Call upon them by name, followed by the words, "Be with me now." Then take a deep breath and imagine that every molecule of oxygen is filled with love, power, and purpose. Let yourself breathe in the fullness of your most capable, empowered essence. You are magic! You can do anything! You are limitless! And most of all, you are doing your very best right now.

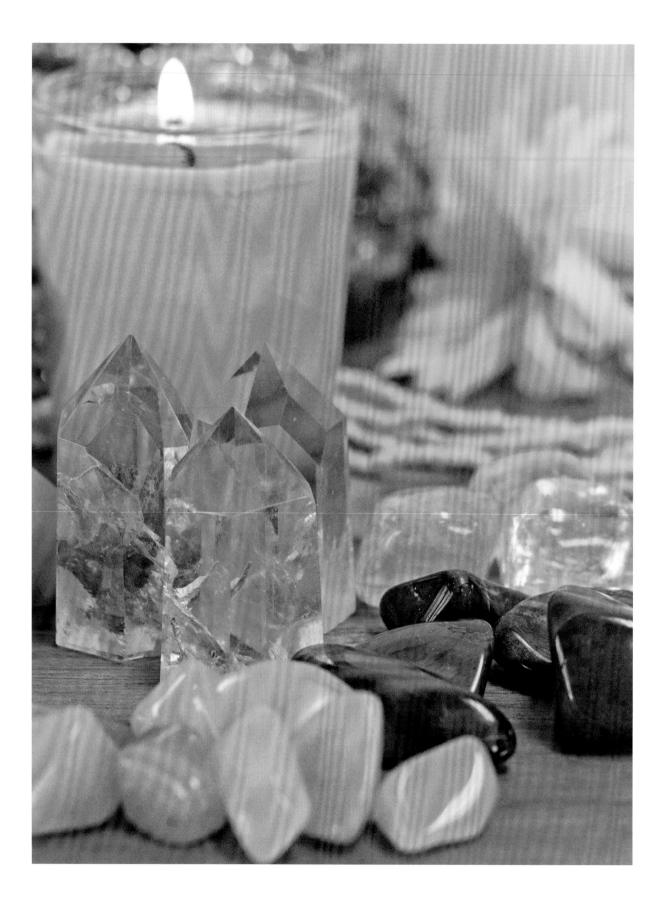

GEMSTONES, ESSENTIAL OILS, AND HERBS OF THE SOLAR PLEXUS CHAKRA

Solar Plexus Gemstones

AMBER will help you channel ancient wisdom, while **TIGER'S EYE** both enhances intuition and activates a protective shield around the bearer. Meditate with it to channel visions of past lives.

CITRINE is bright sunshine captured in time. The primary gemstone for both prosperity and manifestation, citrine opens, aligns, and heals the Solar Plexus Chakra. In China, citrine is called "the Merchant's stone" and is kept in cash registers and cash drawers because it said to attract wealth to the bearer.

GOLDEN HEALER QUARTZ empowers you to locate the internal causes of your own illness and suffering, and also provides you with tools for self-healing. It is also said to magnify prosperity and bring financial abundance.

ORPIMENT is a mineral of instantaneous manifestation, said to more easily manifest thoughts and energies into physical form, accelerating spiritual and physical development.

PYRITE is the gemstone of confidence and inner strength, while **GOLDEN CALCITE** helps you integrate external wisdom. Outside of the United States, pyrite is a well-known talisman of wealth: Gem-grade crystals command top dollar from many collectors.

YELLOW AVENTURINE is the gemstone of fearless adventure and brings empowerment via lived experience. If someone has slighted you, carrying a piece of yellow aventurine can help heal your relationship.

YELLOW FLUORITE is an alternate for citrine, another gemstone of manifestation and wealth. It can also help business owners attract new clients and customers.

YELLOW JADE stimulates the digestive system, helps burn calories, and reduces appetite. Place a piece of yellow jade above the belly button to help ease stomach pain, improve digestion, and increase metabolism.

Consider working with Solar Plexus gemstones at the summer solstice, or any day of the year between noon and 1 p.m. This is when the sun sits at center sky, in its own position of power. The area of the body governed by the Solar Plexus Chakra is the abdomen and intestinal tracts, so if you want to place gems on your body, you can lie down and place them over these areas. This way, your body can conduct the energy of the gems, unifying and connecting them and integrating them into your broader energy field.

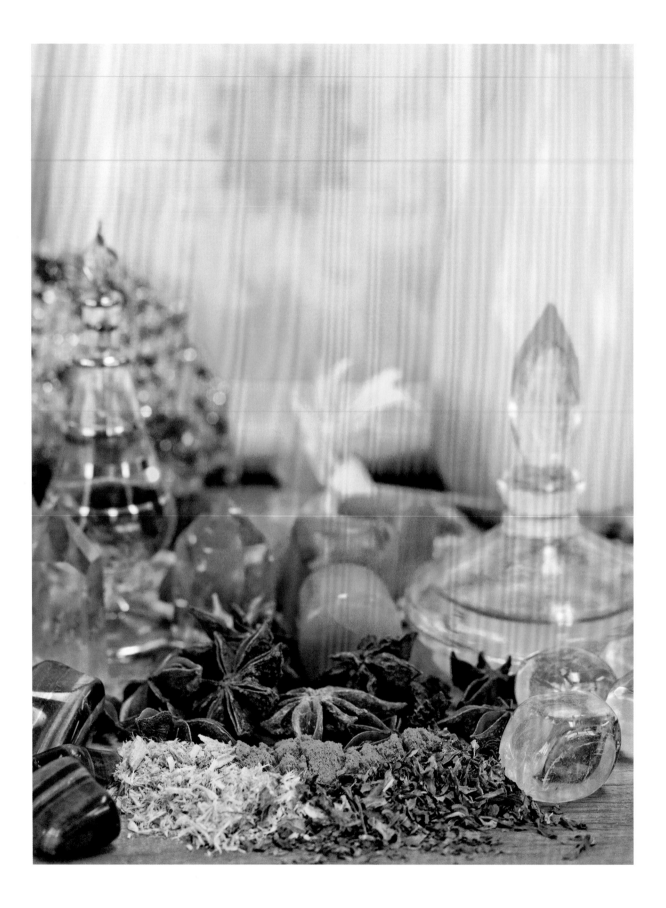

Solar Plexus Herbs
and Essential Oils

Lily of the Valley is the flower of remembrance and sweet recollection, helping you channel the wisdom of your ancestors who have healed and moved into the light. **Lemon** is the fruit of awakening and presence, and helps calm the central nervous system while energizing your power center. **Helichrysum** is an anti-aging ingredient used in high-end skincare lines, but is also an anti-inflammatory, reducing swelling and easing irritation. **Juniper** is a source of protection in particular spaces, helping keep homes and properties safe from theft. **Grapefruit** invigorates and refreshes, while **Neroli** calms frayed nerves and facilitates manifestation. **Tea Tree** is a master healer, because it is anti-bacterial and anti-microbial as well as anti-fungal.

Anise aids in divination and the development of psychic powers, but is also considered a sacred offering to Great Spirit in ritual and ceremony. **Celery** is protective and healing, and **cinnamon** brings prosperity to the bearer. **Marshmallow** enhances clairvoyance, which is the ability to clearly see the future. **Mint** is for luck and wealth, while **Melissa** is useful for love and success magic, and **turmeric** is the world's most powerful antioxidant, the exact color of the Solar Plexus Chakra. **Cumin** is both protective and healing, connecting you with energies of creative expansion. **Copal**, though a resin and not an herb, should be burned when you feel the need for transformation within, or in your spaces. Copal has been used in rites of purification and transformation since Biblical times.

The herbs and resin of the Solar Plexus Chakra can be incorporated into a potent incense blend that, when burned at the full moon, can enhance both personal power and manifestation potential. (It smells amazing, too.)

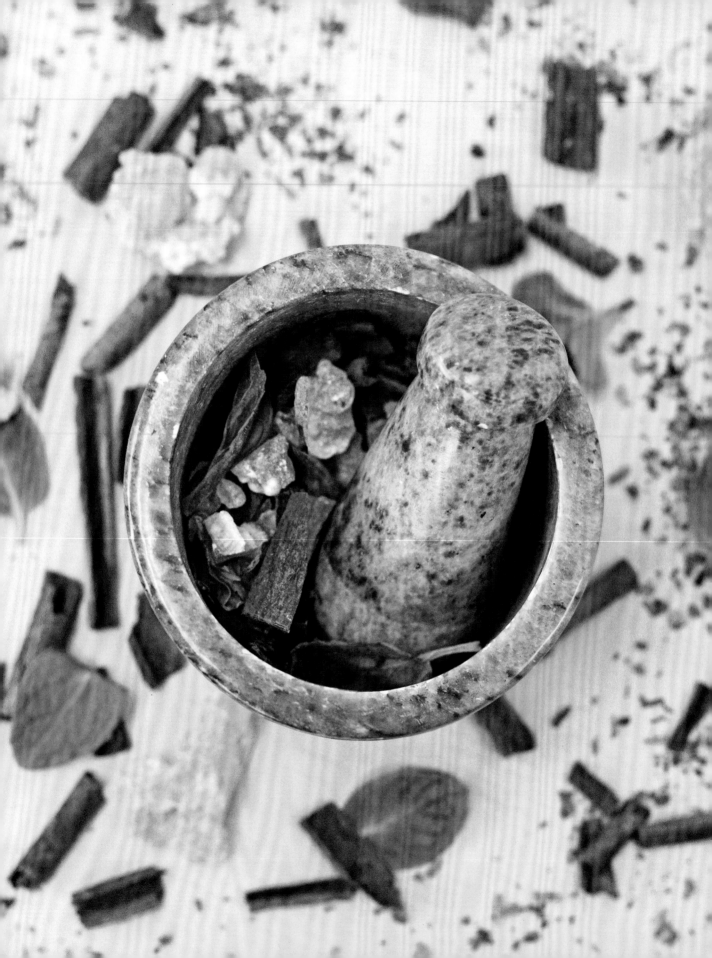

Full Moon Incense Blend for Power and Manifestation

Ingredients

- 1 ounce (28 g) copal resin, ground into powder

- 1 ounce (28 g) mint leaves, crushed

- 1 ounce (28 g) cinnamon bark chips

- 1 ounce (28 g) basil leaves, crushed

- 3 drops each of anise, neroli, and cedar essential oils

Combine all ingredients with a mortar and pestle, grinding until your desired consistency has been reached. Copal clears the space while mint and cinnamon summon energy streams for prosperity. Anise comes through to bless you and seal the energies, while neroli brings blessings and strength. Cedar solidifies your intentions and offers grounding to anchor them. When you burn this Full Moon Incense, you are stepping in the footsteps of your ancestors. Enjoy the experience of connecting to their power, and allow them space to infuse their power into you, blessing you as you carry on their lineage and work in this lifetime. Amen, A'ho, So it is.

Tarot Card, Rune, and Planet of the Solar Plexus Chakra

Major Arcana: The Emperor

In the Major Arcana of the Tarot, The Emperor is the creator and maintainer of sacred structures, both energy-related and within society. In this way, he controls the many ways in which leadership is exercised socially, personally, energetically, and spiritually. While some find The Emperor an imposing figure of control and authority, you might expand your vision of him to include power and possibility. He is a powerful teacher of masculine forms of manifestation and empowerment, a direct line to your own powerful lineage.

Imagine if you were able to access all of your power right now, including power you feel you have lost to relationships and life circumstances. What would it mean to reclaim your deepest sense of power and control? What can you learn from The Emperor's fearless approach to power and leadership?

Rune: Thurisaz

This is one of the most potent of all the runes because it reflects the strength of Thor's mighty hammer, with all its creative and destructive capacities. Thurisaz reminds you that your own power is vast and great. Be respectful of its bounds, and be humble in the face of the power of others around you. Thurisaz reminds you that it is important to find diplomatic solutions to complex problems, reserving Thor's mighty hammer for extreme cases.

How might you bring more compassion to the major challenges of your life, asks Thurisaz, and how might your personal power expand if you could temper it with respect and love for all? Is there a way to align what is best for you with what is best for the whole? When you find yourself in a circumstance where you feel called upon to use strong or excessive force to communicate your opinion or perspective, call upon the energy of this rune to temper your instincts. Save the iron fist for occasions when there are no other options. Even in ancient times of war and conflict, the wise beings in every culture always advised and pursued peace first.

Planet: Sun

The Sun is the main planet corresponding to the Solar Plexus Chakra. This is because, out of all the planets, the Sun has the most direct, linear, and potent energy. The Sun's warmth and strength make it an ideal planetary ally for the work of empowering the soul, helping you access wisdom of objectivity, directness, clarity, decisiveness, and will power.

Archetype of the
Solar Plexus Chakra

In the realm of the Solar Plexus Chakra, **The Father**, **The King**, and **The Queen** are our guides. Each one offers a different perspective on what it means to lead, to love, and to live from a place of empowered wisdom.

The Father teaches us how to love with boundaries, separating the heart from the mind in order to provide limits and structure. The King reminds us that steady and fair rule is more important than reckless decision-making and power plays. The Queen reinforces the role of compassion in leadership, prioritizing the needs of the people and the greater good of the kingdom. Together, they comprise a unified, integrated vision of leadership that is both fair *and* kind. This balance leads toward a future in which all people can feel unified, empowered, and blessed.

Mantra of the
Solar Plexus Chakra

In Sanskrit, *Om Gum Ganapatayei Namaha* is a mantra recited in honor of Lord Ganesha, the Hindu god of obstacle removal and success. Its literal translation is: "I bow to Ganesha, who is capable of removing all obstacles." Recite this mantra when you feel incapable of overcoming the obstacles in front of you, and you will feel Ganesha's power supporting you, and his desire to manifest your success. Remember that obstacles are your teachers: They instruct you to push beyond what you perceive to be your own human limits or potential and explore what is available to you beyond your assumptions. When you encounter an obstacle, observe it, and then dialogue with Ganesha for strategies to circumvent or overcome whatever stands between you and your desires.

Embodiment Exercise:
Solar Plexus Chakra Activation

How do you feel as you reflect on this chapter, which is all about your personal power? Take a moment to acknowledge what an immensely powerful person you are. Use this short meditation to guide you as you activate a deeper sense of personal power in the world.

1/ First, know that your influence is even greater than you can imagine. Think of all the people in the world who have been touched by you over your lifetime. The words you have spoken, the experiences you have shared, the love you have offered—these are your gifts, your legacies. Your energy fingerprint is an extension of you and your impact on the planet. You are a shining star.

2/ Now, consider how it would feel—right here, in this moment—to fully accept and acknowledge your power. How would it be to expect, and even demand, the respect you so richly deserve, and feel it returned to you in every moment, in every relationship, and in every exchange? Imagine the respect and power you desire returning to you from lifetimes past where it may have been lost or released for reasons you no longer remember.

3/ The act of acknowledging that power has been lost and must be returned creates an energy field that can nourish, sustain, and support you. Let that field surround you now, re-assuring you that you are right where you need to be and that your life is unfolding according to a divine plan etched in the bedrock of time. Your power, too, has belonged to you since the dawn of time. You need only claim it now.

4/ As you arrive at this new place of power and possibility, take a deep, cleansing breath and then, like a lion stretching out its paws in the midday sun, let yourself enjoy this moment of centered strength. Imagine that you are like the lion, one of the totem animals of this chakra: You are strong, ferocious, and yet gentle. Once you feel this truth in your bones, seal your knowing with the affirmation, "Amen, A'ho, So it is."

May you be inspired, empowered, and encouraged always. Amen, A'ho, So it is. And on we go.

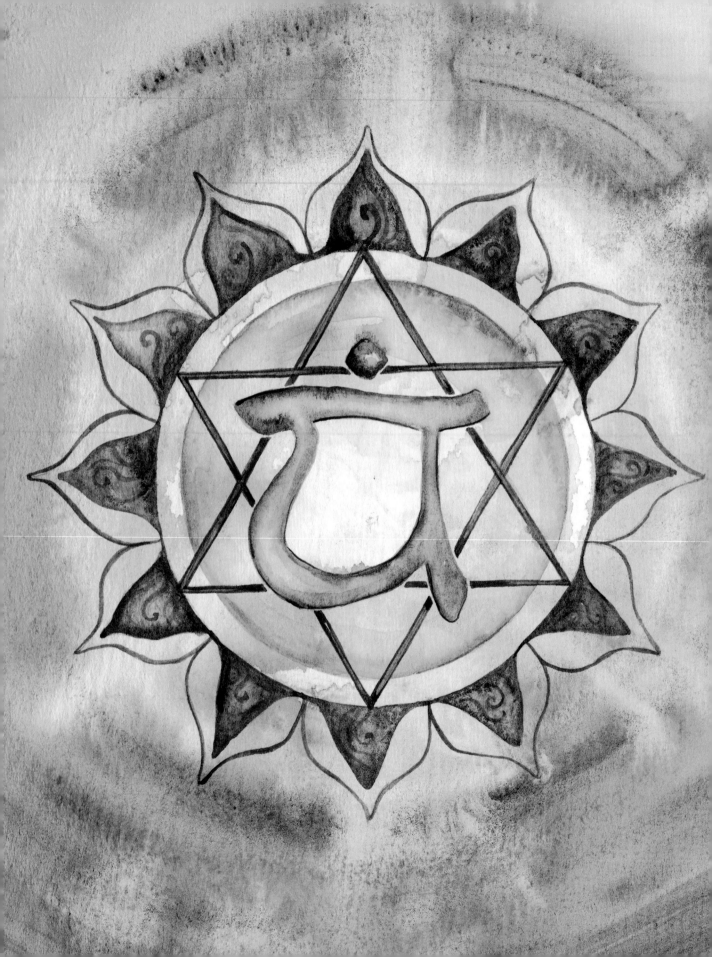

Ch

5

Heart Chakra—

Anahata

The <u>Heart Chakra</u> is the center of your body's energy universe. It sits over your physical heart and regulates energy flow, in the same way that your physical heart regulates the blood flow. Here sits heartache as well as deepest affection; here sits the ability to hold, heal, and help the entire planet, the entire universe; and here sits compassion for all people in all places across time.

When the Heart Chakra is well aligned, you are able to easily and openly love others as you love yourself. When it is blocked, you feel despair, or a lack of hope or optimism. In the realm of love, there are many extremes, from the opposite of love (hate) to the deepest form of love (salvation). Love is the only force in the universe that can actually save you, for it can raise the level of your consciousness to a more elevated state beyond the three-dimensional experience of time and space. Love can also heal the physical body in spontaneous and miraculous ways, since its vibration affects the cells in your body. Indeed, love is the closest one can come to real magic. Love is magic.

Embodiment Exercise:
Heart Chakra Induction

The Heart Chakra induction is designed to open and expand your heart space. Let past hurts go and be fully here now, welcoming the love that surrounds you. Bathe in this awareness as you begin this ritual.

1/ Close your eyes and allow yourself to connect deeply with this moment, noticing the position of your body, the slow inhale and exhale of your breath, the temperature around you. Let go of the stress of yesterday or earlier today, and release your anxiety about what might happen later today or tomorrow. Be here now.

2/ From this place of centered connection, bring your attention to your heart. Cross your hands over your heart, and inhale there. As you exhale, imagine a bright green ray of light emanating from your chest into your hands, surrounding them in a bubble of healing and loving green light. This is the Green or Emerald Ray, the light of love and unconditional, compassionate care that comes only from our heart center. You may already be familiar with the concept of unconditional love, but if not, simply imagine the love you would feel for a baby or small child who needed your help, or a small animal that could not care for itself. That place of unselfish offering is the essence of the Heart Chakra.

3/ Bring your attention to the Green Ray and summon its light into your hands, allowing it to form into a green sphere of healing love energy within your palms. As your hands warm, know that you are holding within them the very energy of love

itself, a powerful tool to be held and used with great care and reverence. Where will you send this Green Ray? To someone you know and love, or to the far corners of the Earth to bless those you have never met? Imagine the possibilities of wielding a beam of healing light energy. In some ways, holding this power is unimaginable—and yet, you already do and always have. By imagining energy, you gather, mold, manifest, and direct it with ease.

4/ Take your hands now and stretch them out before you, sending the Green Ray of light and love to every place it is needed. Ask your guides to send the ray on your behalf where it is needed, trusting that they are aware of spaces in need where you have never been, souls in need you have never met. Let the Love Energy flow through you without restriction, serving as a good channel for its passage. May you be blessed as a conduit of love, always.

5/ Fold your hands in prayer, and then bring your folded hands to your heart space. Give thanks for love within and without: love above, love below. Then close your induction with the universal blessing: Amen, A'ho, So it is."

Reflection Questions for
the Heart Chakra

In Greek, there are many words for love. In fact, in most languages, there are more words for love than there are in English, which can leave us English speakers bereft of language to express our deepest feelings. The four main types of love expressed in the Greek language are *eros*, or romantic love; *filia*, or brotherly love; *storge*, or maternal love; and *agape*, or love for all. Consider these definitions of love and how they might expand your current ideas and definitions of love as you answer the questions that follow.

Brew a cup of rose tea infused with lavender for deep heart-centered peace. Hold a piece of rose quartz, the stone of love, or morganite, which reminds you of your worthiness of love. Then light a pink or green candle, both of which are the colors of the Heart Chakra, as you channel your responses to these prompts:

1/ How has your definition of love changed over the past few years or months, if at all? Does love look different to you today than it has before, and how are you being asked to love differently, or more, than in the past?

2/ Where does love live in your body right now? Ask yourself where in your body you feel most loved and appreciated, and then consider where in your body you need more or deeper love right now. For example, if you are an artist, perhaps you feel that your love is most appreciated in your hands—your creative channels. Or as a mother, especially a mother of a newborn, perhaps you feel most appreciated in your breasts—as channels of milk, a liquid life force. Whichever way you have experienced and received love, consider how you can offer more love to yourself where it is needed today.

3 / Some people in your life may offer you eros, while others bring more filia. Then there is agape, or general love of human-kind. Who are the people in your life that bring each kind of love to you? Take a moment to appreciate them now. Also, be mindful not to expect a different kind of love from people than they are able to offer you, for such is the root of disappointment and sorrow.

When you are ready to close your reflective writing, thank your spirit guides and higher self for attending you while you write and blow out your candles. Store any gems you've used and other writing tools together in a special place so that you'll have them handy when you want to do more reflective writing in the future.

CORRESPONDENCES FOR THE HEART CHAKRA

goddesses

ÁINE, HERA, ISHTAR, QUAN YIN

gemstones

CHRYSOPRASE, GIRASOL, IDOCRASE, MANGANO CALCITE, PINK TOURMALINE, RHODOCHROSITE, ROSE QUARTZ, RUBY

tarot card

MAJOR ARCANA: THE LOVERS

runes

INGWAZ, KENAZ

essential oils/herbs

BERGAMOT, BLACK SPRUCE, CACAO, CARDAMOM, CILANTRO, HAWTHORN BERRIES, JASMINE, LAVENDER, MARJORAM, PALMAROSA, PARSLEY, ROSE, THYME

planet

VENUS

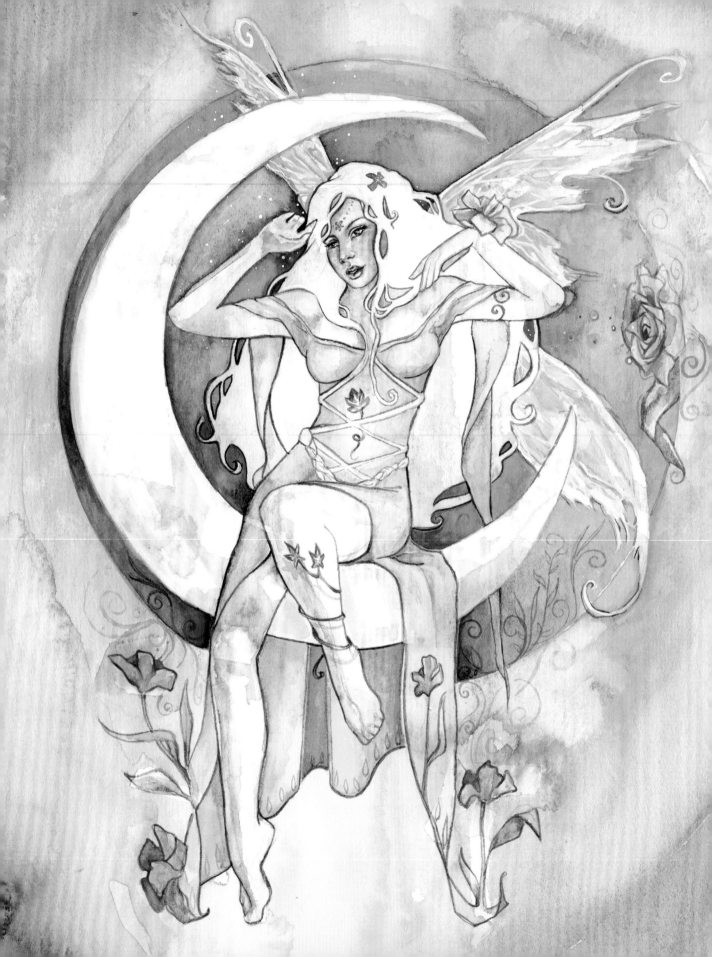

Goddesses of the Heart Chakra

In the same way that there are many names for love around the world, so, too, are there many gods and goddesses of love, each reflecting a different face of this multifaceted energy stream. **Áine** is the Irish/Celtic goddess of wealth, love, and sovereignty or personal integrity. As goddess of both the sun and the moon, she was able to regulate time, as well as beginnings and endings, to help attract new love or to ease suffering when love was lost. **Ishtar** (earlier known as Inanna) was the first true goddess of love from the Akkadian (previously Sumerian) civilization. She revealed the creative and destructive powers of love. As wife to Zeus, the father of the Gods in the Greek pantheon, **Hera** represents another face of love—that of the loyal and dutiful wife, queen of the home domain. Finally, **Quan Yin** offers us yet another perspective on love as pure compassion. She is the bodhisattva of divine feminine mercy and grace.

Each of these goddesses in one way or another is associated with the element of water, which is also the element of the direction of west on the Lakota Medicine Wheel. Quan Yin, for instance, holds a chalice of healing waters that she pours upon the world. Reflect on the power of water to heal, refresh, and renew you. Imagine standing beneath Quan Yin's chalice of healing water, allowing it to flow over and through you. Receive the water from her compassionate stream and commit to carrying its energy into your daily life, pouring it onto others as you have been blessed to receive.

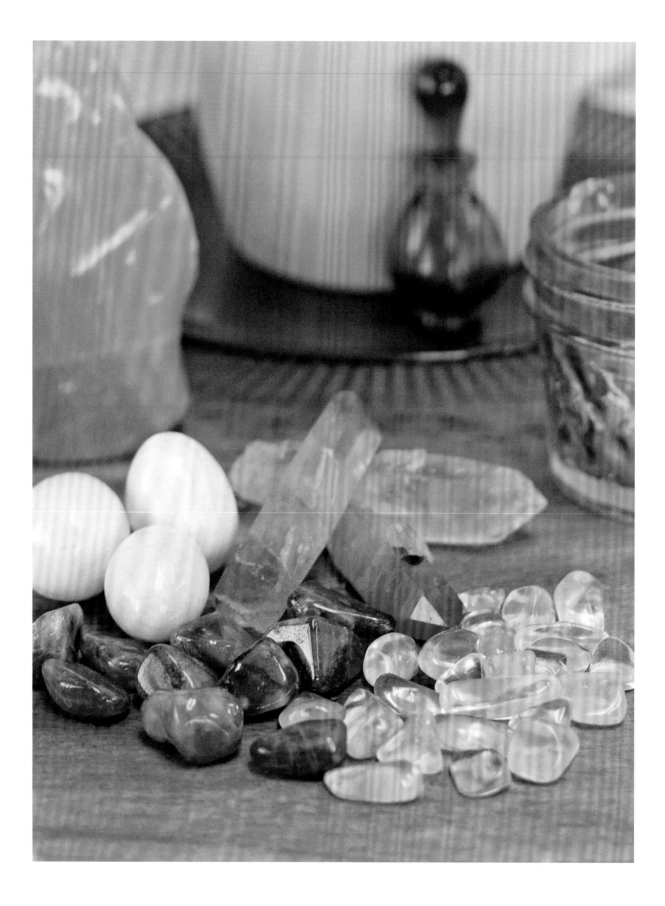

GEMSTONES, ESSENTIAL OILS, AND HERBS OF THE HEART CHAKRA

Heart Chakra Gemstones

PINK TOURMALINE opens the energy stream of unconditional love unlike any other gemstone, while light pink **MANGANO CALCITE** nurses a broken heart back to health. Pink tourmaline reminds you that it is safe to love with an open heart, while mangano calcite heals trauma that has occurred in the heart space before.

ROSE QUARTZ is the primary stone of love, magnifying love both within you and in your home or sacred space. It is known as the mother of all love stones, for it activates universal and unconditional love.

GIRASOL is a lighter and more translucent form of rose quartz, and brings renewal energies to love in your life. Carry it to bring the light of the sun to love in your life.

RHODOCHROSITE is the rose of the Heart Chakra gemstone family, the blooming flower of kindness, love, and possibility. Rhodochrosite brings renewed hope in love. *Rhodo* means "rose" in Greek. When you work with rhodochrosite, imagine holding the rose of love and compassion in your hands. Extend this rose from your hands out into the world, allowing the petals to open and embrace everyone you know and love in the warmth of unconditional acceptance, forgiveness, and peace.

CHRYSOPRASE heals old love wounds and is said to help support cardiac health as well.

IDOCRASE and, to a lesser extent, **RUBY**, bring passion and intensity of physical lust to Heart Chakra work, activating more of the eros-based energies. According to an ancient Indian tale, when a loved one dies, their soul lives on as a ruby in your heart. When you wear ruby jewelry, you honor their legacy.

Try working with your Heart Chakra gemstones by bringing them into your bedroom, which should be a sanctuary of love in your home, whether you are single or in a relationship. Love energies support deep and restful sleep, so anchor your bedroom by placing the stones of love somewhere near its entrance. Even a small table can be transformed into a love altar by draping it in lace or pink velvet and placing intentionally chosen stones from the list above in a shape that is meaningful or inspirational to you.

Consider burning a pink candle each night for five minutes as you transition from day to evening time, releasing cares and anxieties and preparing to shift your thoughts to love and intimate connection. Feel every part of your body soften and open to this intention. Your body, mind, and spirit long for love, as does your environment. Attention and intention, when combined, infuse your space and your spirit with love. Everyone around you will feel and appreciate the efforts you make to deepen and expand love consciousness in your life.

Heart Chakra Herbs and Essential Oils

Hawthorn Berries are the healers of the heart. Protective of both the heart and home, they are able to clear negative stored energy in the Heart Chakra from past pain and heartache. **Jasmine**, grand seductress of the Heart Chakra, tempts lovers with her seductive charms. Few can resist her floral powers of passionate persuasion. **Lavender** is often thought of as a Crown Chakra flower, and of course it can be, but in the heart center, lavender brings peace in love, something many seek but cannot find. **Marjoram** can bring peace and tranquility in love as well, in addition to tranquility in relationships.

Rose is the grand dame of the Heart Chakra, perhaps the most revered of all the love flowers. She guards the door to your heart, while **Thyme** brings healing and purification. **Cilantro** is used in love magic to increase passion. **Parsley** combines passion with fertility, and is excellent for couples when trying to conceive. **Palmarosa** is both a mood and beauty enhancer, aligned with the planet Venus—as many of the Heart Chakra herbs are—to increase its love energies. **Cacao**, a natural aphrodisiac, is used in the sacred Cacao Ceremony to induce love and open the heart channel. Plus cacao eases anxiety and makes you more receptive to love's advances. **Cardamom** adds its lusty spice to any love magic you might conjure, and **Black Spruce** offers cleansing and healing properties to your love rituals. **Bergamot** is a source of clarity in love, helping you see through the rose-tinted glasses of new love to the deeper substance of your attraction.

Consider crafting a love potion to honor the love within your heart that longs to dance with your divine partner. What follows on page 107 is a basic recipe, but feel free to follow *your* heart and add other ingredients as you feel called.

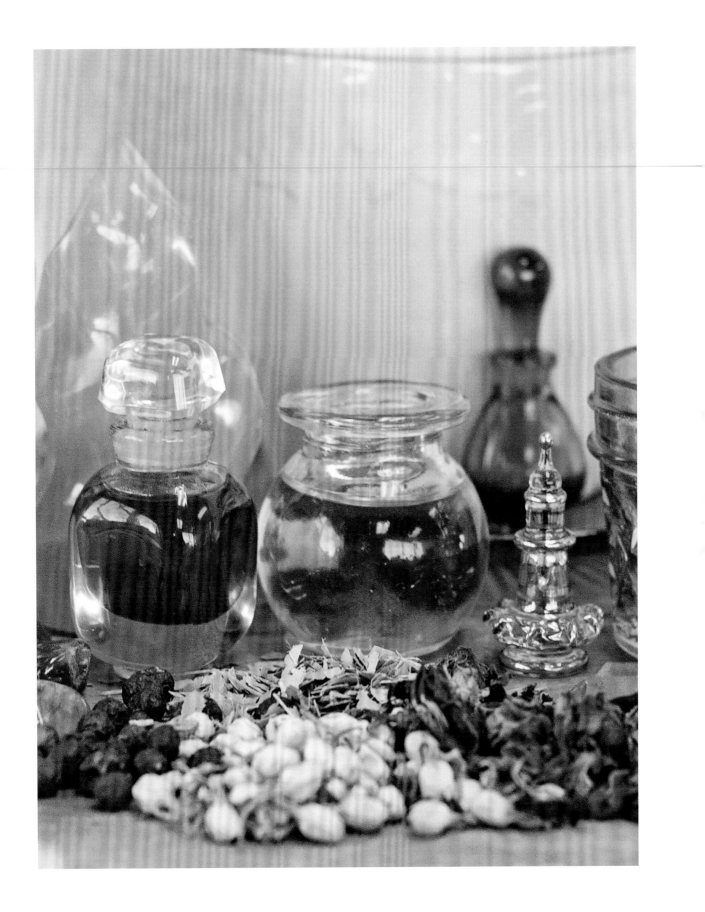

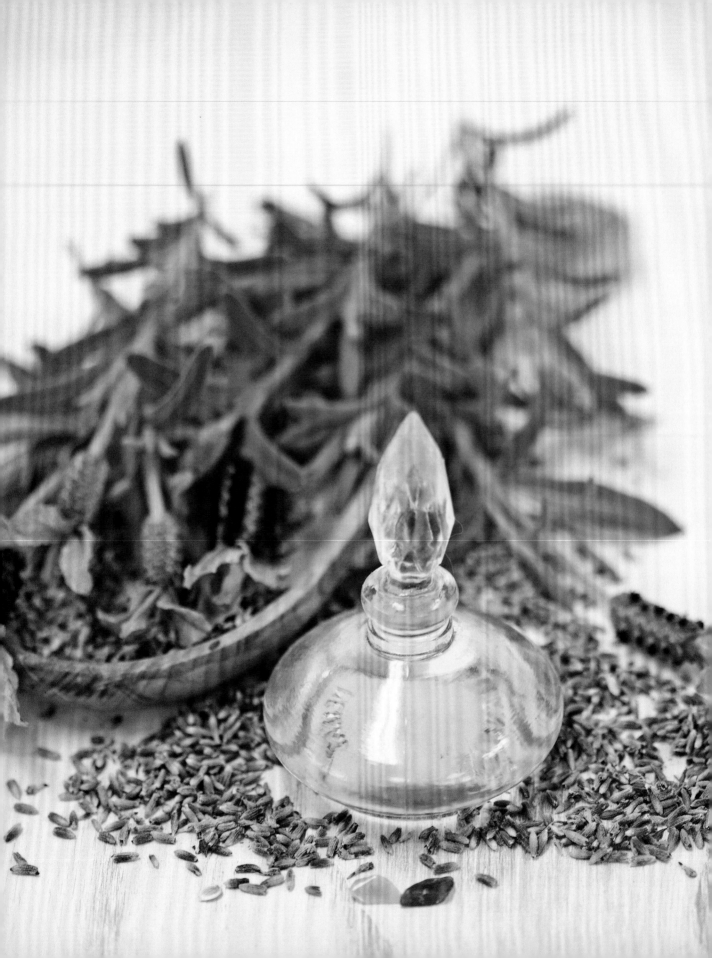

Love's Kiss Perfume to Honor the Sacred Union

Ingredients

- 2 ounces (57 g) carrier oil (Rosehip seed is preferred for this recipe, given its connection to love via rose.)

- 10 drops rose de mai essential oil, for true love's essence

- 2 drops lavender, for peace and balance

- 4 drops ylang tlang, for sexy energies of union and fruition

- 2 drops patchouli, if desired, to ground your energies together in the dance of love

- 2 chip stones, 1 each of rose quartz for love and emerald for fidelity (or substitute ruby for passion or chrysoprase for healing)

Gently combine all the ingredients, asking your Love Guides—the light beings who guide you as you engage in human relationships—to attend the process and bless your desired union. Call upon Venus, too, to bless you with love, beauty, and desire now and as you wear this potion. Amen, A'ho, So it is.

Tarot Card, Runes, and Planet
of the Heart Chakra

Major Arcana: The Lovers

In the Major Arcana of the tarot, The Lovers represent both a physical partnership as well as the idea of union, or a choice between one lover and another. When you work with the energy of this card, ask yourself what you *really* desire. List the qualities you seek in a partner. Create an image in your mind of what life will be like for you in love, right down to the finest detail. The Lovers card invites you to dream big and wide, setting an intention for love that may be more expansive than you have imagined in the past. Remember that when you are in partnership and set the intention for expansion in love, you are also bringing your partner with you into this new level of awareness. Be gentle and mindful, and always ask that the highest good unfolds for all beings.

Runes: Kenaz and Ingwaz

Kenaz is the rune of romantic and erotic love, physical partnership, and procreation, while Ingwaz is the home of "storge," familial love, and the love of home. One pulls you into relationship with another—the physical expression of desire—while the other pulls you out of relationship to express love to those around you as well as within your physical spaces—perhaps through adornment and decoration, as well as creation and dedication of unique altar spaces. The balance of Kenaz and Ingwaz brings internal and external love energies. Meditate on these divergent messages of love to understand where in your life you need to connect with one or the other, or both.

Planet: Venus

Venus is the ultimate planet of love and beauty. In astrology, your placement of Venus represents the way you love yourself and others. Venus represents your youthfulness and vitality, as well as your capacity for love—both of self and others. Ask yourself: Where in your heart do you need to allow more love to bloom? Call upon Venus to soften your heart and to allow it to be more available to those who want to love you. If you are looking for love, call upon Venus to attract new love to you.

Archetype of the Heart Chakra

In the realm of the Heart Chakra, three archetypes emerge, all of which represent a sacred duality that can be expressed in the form of two physical lovers, or within one person as the balance of Divine Masculine and Divine Feminine.

The Lovers represent the dual expression of love: the feminine softness of understanding and safety combined with masculine strength and power. Together, The Lovers reflect your own duality and ability to be both tender and strong, soft and protective. **The Soulmates** represent the earthly duo of lovers who are fated to meet, regardless of the physical or emotional distance that separates them. It is said that every soul incarnated in physical form will meet at least one soulmate to whom he or she will be undeniably attracted. Your soulmate represents the completion of your soul in another human form. **The Twin Flame** is your other half in spirit form who safeguards, protects, and loves you from above, but never incarnates during your lifetime. All souls have a mirror energy on the other side: Many people have "met" their Twin Flame in spirit form, and appreciate having a partner soul in spirit form looking after them from the spirit realm. (To meet such a spirit, simply call upon your love guides and tell them you are ready to encounter your twin spirit. Most often, this encounter happens in dream time. For many, encountering the twin in dream state has reduced physical challenges like insomnia.) It's like having your own guardian angel who knows you better than anyone else—after all, he or she is your other half!

Mantra of the
Heart Chakra

Jai Radha Madhav is a mantra that celebrates the divine love between Radha and Krishna. In many ways, their love is a physical representation of a spiritual union, one in which the individual is able to love and celebrate the collective, and vice versa. They were unable to be together—Radha was married, Krishna was king—but they were true soulmates, connected by their thoughts and their essence across space and time. They represent the power of true love to defy all constraints. If you have ever experienced a soul connection that was blocked by obstacles you thought you could not overcome, you already know the essence of this mantra, which exalts the triumph of soul connection despite impediments.

Embodiment Exercise:
Heart Chakra Activation

The purpose of the Heart Chakra activation is to help you have a physical experience of love energy. Once your body registers the vibration of love on the physical plane, it becomes far easier to tap into this energy in the future. Let this meditation guide you.

1/ Reflect for a moment on your deepest experience of love in this lifetime—the experience in which you felt most seen, most valued, most appreciated, most nourished, and most accepted for who you truly are. How did you feel? Specifically, how did your body feel? How did your spirit feel? How did your energy field feel to you then: Was it alive, vital, and full of possibility? How was your self-esteem at that time? How did you think of yourself?

2/ When you are in a state of love, a whole new world of opportunity opens to you. Love is the most powerful energy force in our universe, and with its power you can create whatever you seek, heal your body, and experience a profound level of joy. All you have to do is receive. Love is a gift that constantly desires to be received. Say yes. It is safe to say yes to love.

3/ Imagine a green tidal wave of love energy washing over your whole body, filling you with a deep sense of purpose and peace, knowing that you are loved by beings seen and unseen. You are held by a legion of angels and ancestors who know, love, see, and appreciate you.

4/ Next, bring that love energy to your physical heartspace, placing your hands over your heart. If there are pockets or places within you that still feel heavy with the traumas of the past, send extra love energy there. Remind the little girl or little boy within you that you are here now, and she or he is safe. Remind the little girl or little boy within that all is well now, and you are able to offer her or him whatever is needed to heal the past in this moment. Feel her or him receive the love now that has been missing, filling the holes and gaps with the Green Ray of healed love.

5/ From this place of healed wholeness, you can emerge now, renewed and ready to seek and speak your truth. Take a deep breath here, accepting and allowing love and truth to rest within your spirit. On the exhale, let go of any hesitation or anxiety. Know that you are worthy of this love: Receive it, enjoy it, and spread it into the world.

May you be loved, held, and blessed always. Amen, A'ho, So it is. And on we go.

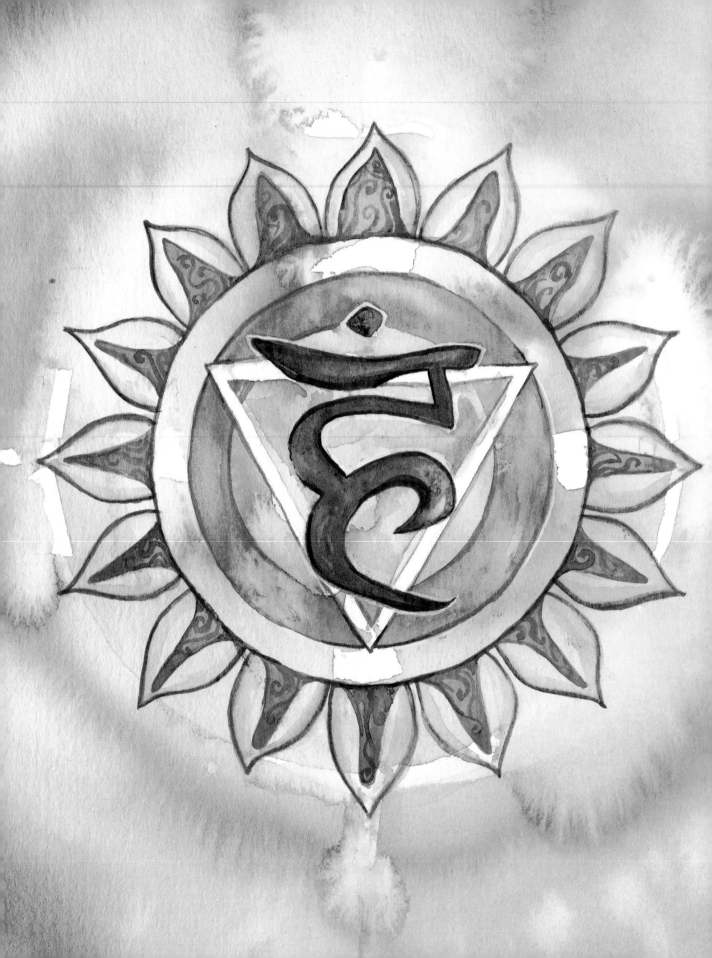

Ch

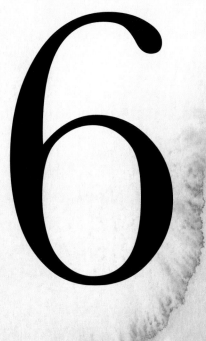

6

Throat Chakra—
Vishuddha

How do you feel about truth? In this chapter, truth is the operative word, while voice is its secondary focus. At the <u>Throat Chakra</u>, many people focus on voice and speech—that is, your ability to articulate thoughts and ideas. What is most important at the Throat Chakra is not *how* you communicate, but *what* you communicate. The "what" is your truth, your deepest wisdom; the "how" is your channel for sharing your truth. Both the "what" and "how" of truth sit here at the Throat Chakra, which is located at the center of your physical throat (or your Adam's apple).

How do you define "truth"? Some say truth is a personal quest to understand the values and beliefs that guide your life choices and decisions. Others suggest that there is a collective truth, a unified wisdom all can aspire to and seek to integrate. Let the intersection of these two approaches inspire you to explore individual and collective truths, using your gift of discernment to understand how to integrate what you see, learn, and experience into your life.

Embodiment Exercise:
Throat Chakra Induction

The Throat Chakra holds the sum total of your lived experiences with voice, expression, and truth. Many people find that exploring this chakra is complicated because they were silenced or repressed in childhood. Think of the myth of the "perfect child" who only speaks when spoken to. You may not have lived this experience, but those who did now have an opportunity to heal the silenced child within whose voice was not welcomed, sought, or appreciated.

Perhaps your experience with truth and voice is different. Perhaps your voice has always been sought and appreciated, or perhaps you were encouraged to speak your truth as a child, but now, as an adult, you feel silenced—at work, socially, or within your family. Whatever your experience, you can use this meditation to guide your exploration of the Throat Chakra.

1 / First, bring your attention to the present moment and take a deep breath. Now, bring your attention to your throat, and swallow as deeply and intentionally as you can. (When you swallow, you regenerate the energies around your Throat Chakra. Anytime you feel lost for words or unable to articulate your needs, swallow and soften your neck.)

2 / Ask yourself, "What is my deepest truth?" Allow yourself a moment to answer. Yes, it's a big—even overwhelming—question, but it is one you can use to move more fully into your soul's intended purpose. Understanding and articulating your personal truth is the first step in acknowledging what you need to feel more fully alive.

3 / As an answer comes to you, simply sit with it. Feel into it. Inhabit and experience it in your body. Once you understand your deepest personal truths, other truths will open from there. For example, if your deepest personal truth is that energy is real, then other truths emerge: If energy is real, magic is real; if magic is real, anything is possible; if anything is possible, you are limitless; if you are limitless, your wildest dreams can come true.

4 / Dream free, dear one. Know that you are treasured beyond measure and trust that you are expressing yourself in service of the highest truth of All Beings. Let the peace of your inner truth surround you.

5 / When you feel connected to truth on every level, ask your ancestors and spirit guides to be with you as you integrate what you have seen. Welcome their presence as they surround you. They are here to help you love and honor yourself more deeply than ever before. When you feel fully wrapped in this blanket of support and wisdom, close your induction with the universal blessing: Amen, A'ho, So it is.

May you be comforted by the presence of your inner truth, always.

Reflection Questions for
the Throat Chakra

Ancient Romans coined a famous phrase: *In vino veritas* or "In wine, truth." They believed that a person's truth emerges primarily when inebriated, or when she or he is allowed to expand his or her awareness beyond the present moment, beyond the veil and filter of time, space, convention, and expectation. But you don't need to consume alcohol in order to do this. Ask yourself: If you could drink a glass of virtual wine right now, what truths would spill from your lips? If you felt free to express yourself without fear of repercussion, what would you say, and to whom?

Consider working with amazonite, which is often referred to as the primary gem of the Throat Chakra. Hold it in your right hand, which is your feminine, receptive hand, and feel its energy rise and flow through your body. Brew yourself a hot cup of geranium and lemongrass tea, or steep mulling herbs, such as cloves, cinnamon, and orange, with a rich Cabernet, and sip slowly as you meditate upon the following questions:

1/ Letting go of fear and hesitation as you consider your response, who in your life most needs to hear your truth? Keep in mind that the person who most needs to hear your truth is often *you*. The person who most needs to hear your truth may also be deceased. That is no obstacle. Speak your truth anyway. The dead can hear you.

2/ Are you keeping secrets in your life, and, if so, from whom? When you think about secrets, how do you feel? Anxious, heavy, and weighed-down, perhaps? If you carry such secrets, where in your life can you release them or set them down?

3/ Who in your life most honors your truth—your most authentic and honest self? How does the honoring of your truth make you feel? Who might benefit if you could pay this gift forward?

When you are ready to close your reflective writing, thank your spirit guides and higher self for attending you while you write, and blow out your candles. Store any gems you've used and other writing tools together in a special place so that you'll have them handy when you want to do more reflective writing in the future.

CORRESPONDENCES FOR THE THROAT CHAKRA

goddesses

ALETHEIA, VERITAS

gemstones

AMAZONITE, ANGELITE, AQUA AURA QUARTZ, CELESTITE, TURQUOISE

tarot cards

MAJOR ARCANA: JUSTICE AND JUDGMENT

rune

ANSUZ

essential oils/herbs

BAY LAUREL, BLACKBERRY, BLUE CHAMOMILE, BLUE YARROW, COLTSFOOT, COMMON SAGE, ELDERBERRY, EUCALYPTUS, FIR BALSAM, GERANIUM, LEMONGRASS, PETITGRAIN, PERU BALSAM

planet

MERCURY

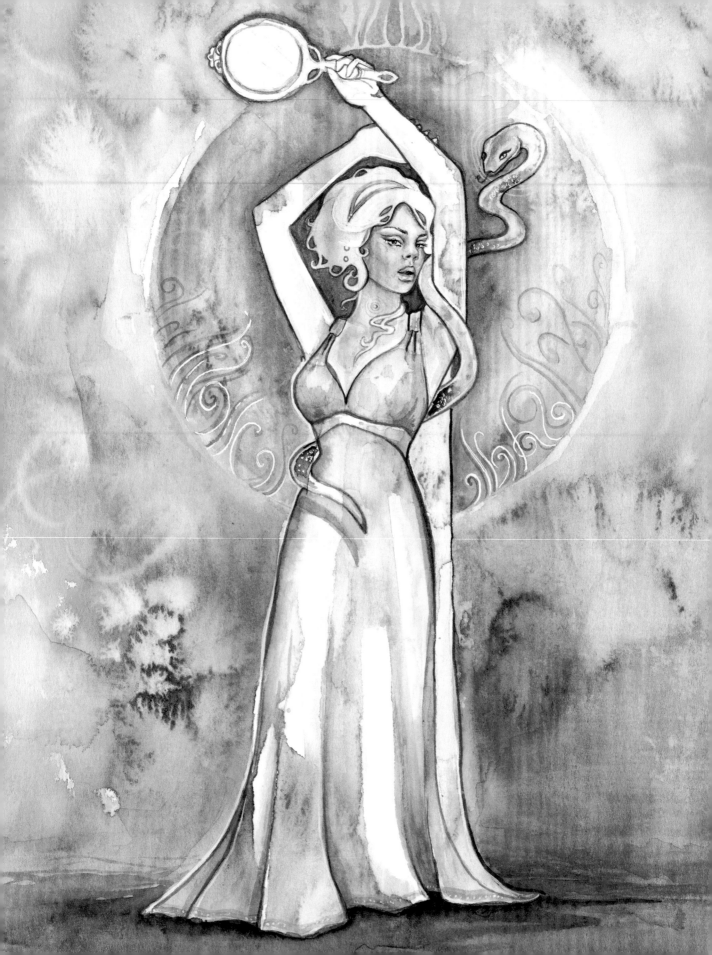

Goddesses of the Throat Chakra

Two goddesses offer themselves for work on the Throat Chakra, where the voice of power emerges. **Veritas**, in Roman mythology, is the daughter of Chronos, the god of time. She is goddess of Truth—with a capital T—and has access to the Truth of the past, present, and future. Through her access to All Truth, she becomes an oracle, a seer of what lies ahead and a clarifier of what lies behind. Veritas reveals the connection between truth (the Throat Chakra) and insight (the Third Eye Chakra), and thus serves as a sacred bridge between these two energy centers.

Aletheia is the ancient Greek goddess of truth and remembrance and is Veritas's counterpart in the Greek pantheon. In Greek, *Aletheia* literally means "not hiding" or "not hidden," reflecting the parts of ourselves that need liberation. However, where Veritas sees the literal, Aletheia is capable of seeing the figurative; in her realm, shades of gray exist between the extremes of black and white. So it is with your truth: Somewhere between right and wrong are layers of depth and opacity that are worthy of exploration.

To work with these goddesses, simply call upon them by name and ask them to pull back any layers of illusion in your life, offering you unfettered access to complete truth so that you can live in the light of clarity. Amen, A'ho, So it is.

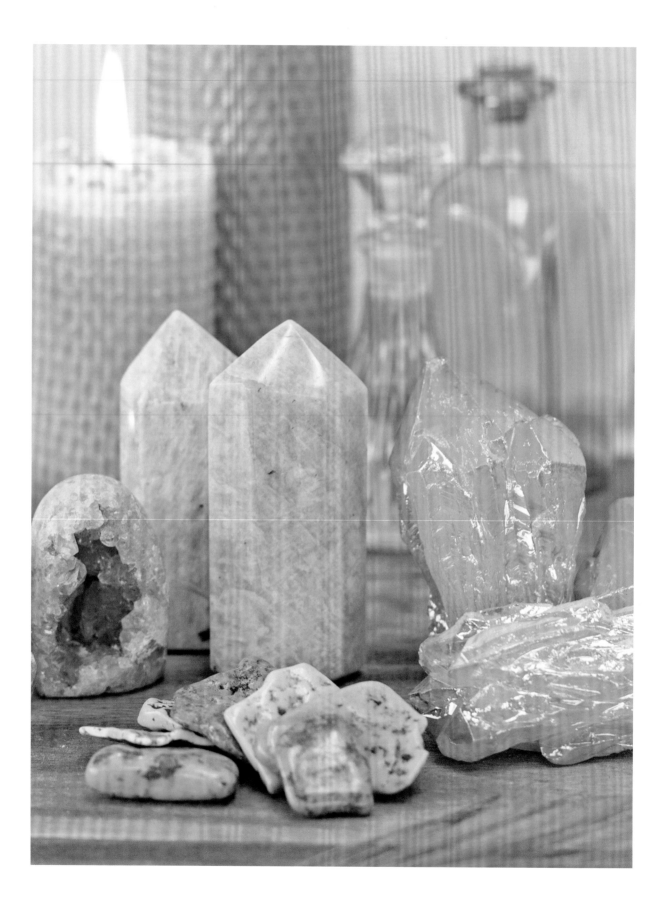

GEMSTONES, ESSENTIAL OILS, AND HERBS OF THE THROAT CHAKRA

Throat Chakra Gemstones

The gems of this chakra are thought to be the gems of Lemuria, an ancient civilization associated with the dolphin kingdom, and represent wisdom that was encrypted and stored in crystals before that civilization's collapse. **AQUA AURA QUARTZ**, one of the primary Lemurian gemstones, is a strong purifier of the aura, and also promotes strength, tenacity, and prosperity.

AMAZONITE is the primary stone of truth, and boosts confidence for public speakers, helping them articulate even the most difficult words and subjects with ease.

ANGELITE (in crystalline form, known as **CELESTITE**) invokes the angelic realms to attract the presence of angels, including archangels, in your spaces. Carry this gem with you or sleep near it in order to feel more connected to your own personal angels and guides.

TURQUOISE has been revered for centuries among Native Americans who consider it a potent purifier and healer, as well as a stone that strengthens and protects warriors in battle. In ancient Persia, it was revered as a source of good fortune.

Connect with your Throat Chakra gemstones during times of fear or confusion. Here's how to do this: Lie down in a comfortable position and hold one to three of your favorite light blue Throat Chakra stones in your right hand, the Receiving Hand, through which energy enters your body. (Some people feel their left hand is their Receiving Hand; go with what feels right for you.) Set the intention to receive peace, wisdom, and truth, which are the gifts of the Throat Chakra. Then transfer the stones to your left, or Projecting Hand, so that you can send this energy out into the world as a blessing for all. Imagine beaming a bright blue ray of truth and light out into the world for all to see, receive, and enjoy.

Then, place one of the Throat Chakra stones on the center of your throat, and allow yourself to receive the Blue Ray of truth through its vibrational healing pattern. Finally, become mindful of your saliva, the vehicle of your life force energy anchored in the Throat Chakra. Swallow deeply from this place of illuminated truth, connecting to your own center of spoken wisdom. Trust this wisdom; it is your deepest knowing, inherited over time and tested by experience, both yours and your ancestors. May it serve you well.

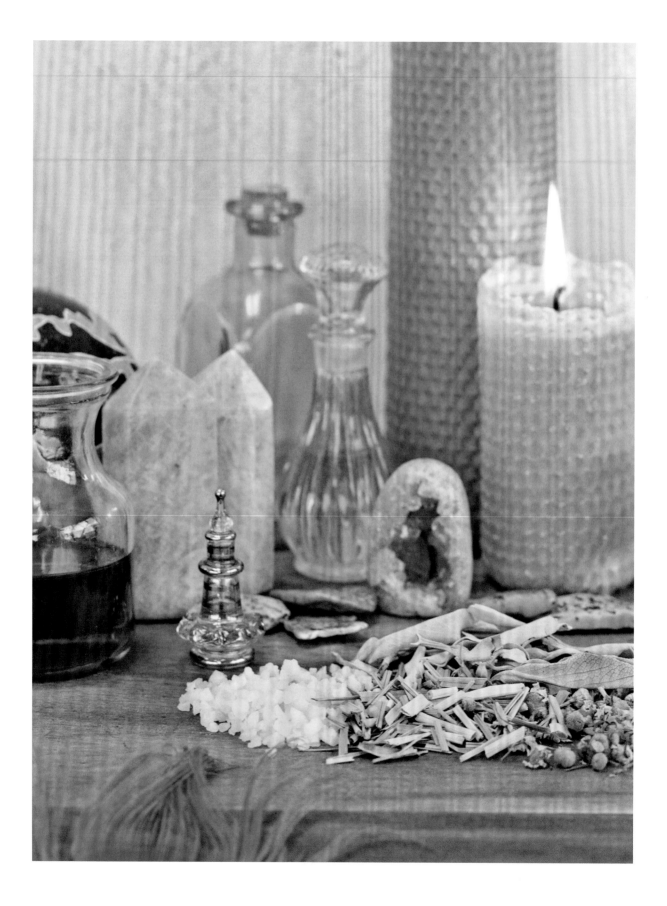

Throat Chakra Herbs
and Essential Oils

Coltsfoot brings love and psychic visions, while **Blackberry** offers protection and prosperity to the bearer. **Elderberry** protects the bearer from physical harm and is a master healer. **Common Sage** is best for healing and grounding, and **Lemongrass** heals a broken heart. **Bay Laurel** brings psychic power, and **Eucalyptus** is cleansing, uplifting, and healing on all levels. **Petitgrain** is calming and helps ensure a good night's rest when blended with lavender and **Blue Chamomile**, another essential oil known to soothe frayed nerves and calm a nervous mind. **Blue Yarrow** brings water element energy to clear stuck energy and repairs the aura while **Peru Balsam** helps deepen meditation and aligns your chakra system. **Fir Balsam** grounds you deeply in the forests of grandfather trees, easing worries and concerns and helping you to be fully present in the moment.

A beautiful way to work with these herbs and essential oils is to make an incense or perfume called The Peace of Truth. Have you noticed how peace arrives when you are centered in your personal truth, your attention anchored in the present moment? It is so easy to worry about the past or future instead of allowing yourself to connect with the joy of right here, right now. In these moments, remember how futile worry is. Nothing you worry about can be changed by your worry; and, in fact, the things you fear can manifest if you send too much energy their way. So, simply be here, now.

This simple but very effective recipe on page 125 shows you how to craft an incense blend to help you make a scent association with this concept of mindful presence.

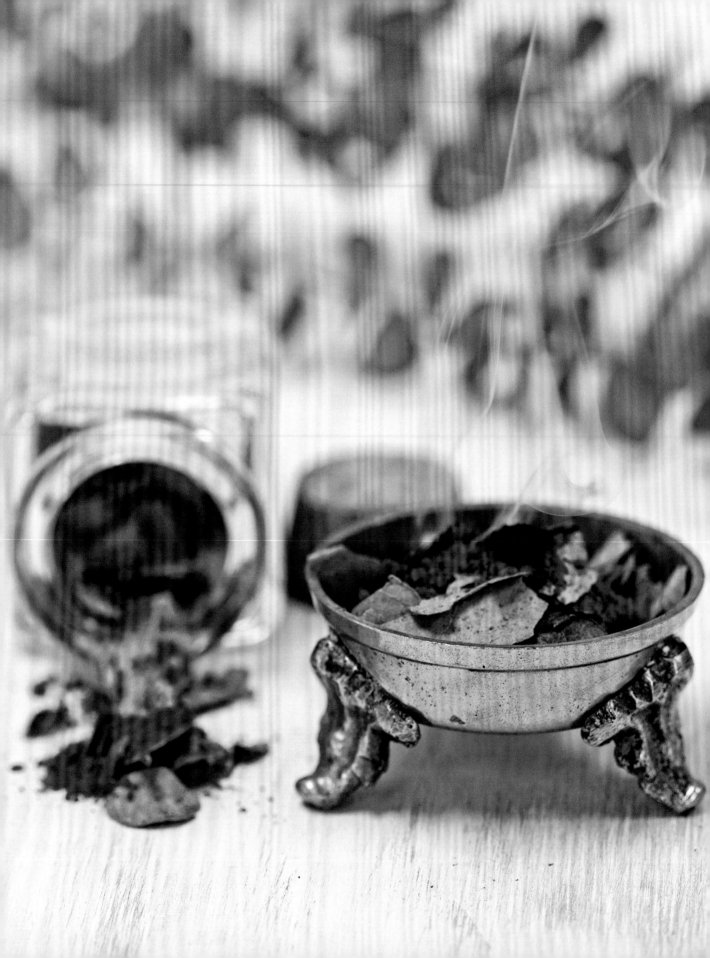

The Peace of Truth
Incense Blend

Ingredients

- 1 ounce (28 g) dried eucalyptus leaves, crushed

- 1 ounce (28 g) bay laurel leaves, crushed

- 1 ounce (28 g) sandalwood powder

- 3 drops each of petitgrain, Peru balsam, and fir balsam essential oils or absolutes

Combine all the ingredients with a mortar and pestle until your desired consistency is reached. Whisper prayers of peace into your blend as you grind, and blow your breath, your sacred life force, into the ingredients. When you are finished, add a small chip stone of a resonant gemstone or mineral, and then store the mixture in a tightly sealed jar until ready to burn on a charcoal disk. Whenever you burn this blend, receive the peace of its ingredients with gratitude. Allow them to uplift and bless you. Amen, A'ho, So it is.

Tarot Cards, Rune, and Planet of the Throat Chakra

Major Arcana: Justice and Judgment

In Tarot, Justice and Judgment are two very different cards—one is mundane, the other spiritual in nature. Justice represents outcomes, decisions, and matters of judgment in the mortal realm. In the Major Arcana, it is reflective of legal process, at times, as well as one's own personal inclination or temptation to judge others. The Judgment card reflects a higher calling to truth, and a higher order of accountability than we find on the mortal level. There, judgment reflects the possibility of rebirth through reflection and redemption. Both are accountings of right and wrong, but their scope is by nature different. One calls you to look down and out, across your life and your decisions. Where can your personal judgment be enhanced or improved? The other asks you to look up and across, to the span of the universe, to listen for signs and heed the call of your soul. Your transformation is at hand, and at its core is your truth. Truth may either inspire your rebirth or facilitate it; either way, these cards are both strong signs that your soul is in a state of evolution.

Rune: Ansuz

Ansuz is the rune of clear communication and transmission of information, as well as the rune of truth, although the way Ansuz expresses truth is through wisdom. Ansuz is one of the primary runes associated with Odin himself, King of the Norse pantheon and father of the runic system, which he downloaded during a nine-day journey in the forest where—suspended from the Tree of Knowledge—he received the runes and their meanings as guidance for his path and teachings. Meditate on this rune to understand how to align truth and communication in your life.

Planet: Mercury

Mercury is the planet of communication and the messenger of the solar system. In Greek mythology, Mercury was the messenger to the gods, swiftly delivering important news and messages to them from Mount Olympus. When Mercury is direct, communication on Earth is swift and easy, with fewer chances for miscommunication; however, when Mercury reverses its forward movement and turns retrograde, which happens twice each year, be mindful of chances for miscommunication. It is best not to sign contracts or formalize business dealings when Mercury is retrograde. Knowing what sign Mercury is in within your own natal chart can help you understand better how you prefer to communicate, which in turn can help you articulate and speak your truth more effectively.

Archetypes of the
Throat Chakra

There are many potential archetypes of truth. It is not surprising that such a powerful concept should have so many human faces and incarnations. Still, two main archetypes, **The Guru** and **The Seeker**, represent common embodiments of Throat Chakra energies. In Sanskrit, the word *guru* refers to the path from ignorance to enlightenment; thus, any teacher, any person, any being who en-lightens you with wisdom and insight that deepens your spiritual understanding is a guru. For some, the activation of the Throat Chakra leads to ascension and enlightenment, as well as the call to share that enlightenment with others. That is The Guru's journey.

The Seeker is another truth and wisdom archetype that takes the role of student instead of teacher. The Seeker simply enjoys the archaeology of learning and experience for its own sake, and for the sake of personal development, while The Guru takes her truth and wisdom to a place of teaching and sharing, for the enlightenment of others. Both are valid and important.

Mantra of the
Throat Chakra

Om Kumara Kushalo Dayayei Namaha is a Sanskrit mantra and blessing that means, "Salutations to the divine mother, who brings blessings to children." You are indeed a child of Gaia, and as you connect with your truth at the Throat Chakra, you become more capable of locating and speaking truth. This process of individuation, rooted in psychoanalysis, simultaneously separates you from the Mother and links you back more directly to her.

Kumara means "child" in Sanskrit, but it also means "challenging mortality," and is a reminder that truth and wisdom are the gifts and challenges of living a mortal life. The more wisdom gathered, the more ease becomes possible; and yet the more wisdom gathered, the more difficult it can be to trust in the Divine. This mantra is an invitation for you to acknowledge how far you have come in your personal spiritual journey and how many gifts you have received along the path. As you meditate with this mantra, ask yourself how truth and wisdom have blessed you, and give thanks for these blessings.

Embodiment Exercise:
Throat Chakra Activation

Throat Chakra activation is about articulating and embodying your deepest inner truth. Truth is such an ambiguous concept: In order to activate it in your life and embody it fully, you must ask yourself what truth means to you. What is *your* truth? Closely linked to truth is power, and, of course, love; in fact, the adjacent chakras to your Throat Chakra are the Heart Chakra and Solar Plexus, as well as the Third Eye, or center of your intuition. All are intimately connected, as they comprise our different ways of knowing and seeing. Let this meditation guide you as you activate your Throat Chakra.

1/ Be aware that activating the truth center of your energy field is a complex feat—but at the same time, it is the easiest decision you will ever make. Are you ready to stand in your truth? Are you ready to show up fully and authentically in your life and take responsibility for your words, actions, and intentions? If you answer yes to these questions, your Throat Chakra is already open and active.

2/ Next, trust that you are safe to express your truth to whomever needs to hear it, and whenever and in whatever way it needs to be communicated. Ask for support from your spirit guides and the goddesses of truth, Veritas and Aletheia, as you step fully into your truth and use your voice to express your truth in the world.

3/ To do this, invoke the bright blue essence of the Blue Ray of light. Imagine this light emanating from your throat, the center of your activated truth, and imagine sending that beam of blue light out from your Throat Chakra to the very center of the universe, where it can connect to other beams of truth light-energy and reflect the radiance of collective truth back to you and back to our planet—back to all of the trees and flowers, animals, and bodies of water. Truth is where souls connect most powerfully. Next to love, truth is the most powerful energy vibration.

4/ Once you find and connect to truth in your life, stay there for as long as it feels right to you. Let truth envelop you and nourish and support you. You are the child of truth, and so truth is your sacred birthright. Imagine radiating this truth out into the world. Think about ways you can bring this truth forward in your own life, mirroring it to those around you.

5/ Finally—and most importantly—think about how you can bring this truth forward for your personal good, to help you evolve, develop, and grow. This is your time to become and expand, anchoring your actions in your authentic inner knowing. Enjoy this phase of your soul's development, for it is here you find your greatest compass and True North.

May you walk in truth and beauty, always. Amen, A'ho, So it is. And on we go.

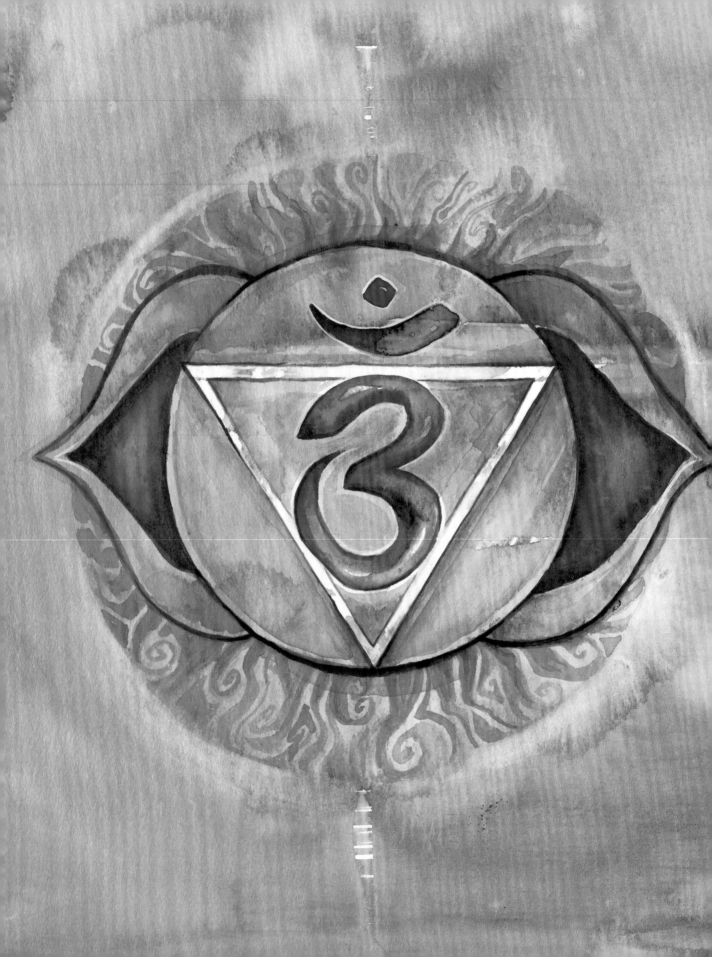

Ch

7

Third Eye Chakra—

Ajna

The Third Eye Chakra is the seat of intuition and the clarities intuition brings. When your Third Eye is open and activated, you become an energy peacock: You have many "eyes" that see the world in full, vibrant color, and all of your senses are available to you as sources of wisdom and information. When your Third Eye is blocked, however, you feel the opposite: unclear, unfocused, and unable to sense what is happening around you.

It is possible to learn, live, and thrive either way; in fact, many people function quite well without an active, open Third Eye Chakra. So, what might lead someone to work on her intuition and actively seek to open and activate the Third Eye? Often, a sense of despair and dissatisfaction. The most common question people ask when they reach their thirties, forties, and fifties is, "Is this all there is to life?" When you begin to seek to understand the depths of life, death, consciousness, and reality in this way, you will know you are ready to work closely with the Third Eye Chakra, through which you can develop enhanced vision and insight. Here, there are no boundaries. Here, wisdom can and does come to you from all directions. Here, you can see clearly and vividly. Thus, the question becomes: What will you do with what you learn?

Embodiment Exercise:

Third Eye Chakra Induction

The purpose of this induction is to help you distinguish your spirit sight from your physical sight. Intuition can be tricky, because many people have not yet learned to fully trust what they cannot see with their human eyes. But intuition is not so much about seeing as it is about sensing. So, to help you connect with your Third Eye Chakra, I will ask you to close your seeing, human eyes, because they will not always be accurate guides while exploring the deeper terrain of consciousness and awareness. Take your time here: This is the final frontier of metaphysical and spiritual development. Once you trust that you can receive and retrieve wisdom from non-local sources not bound by the constraints of space and time, the entire experience of your life can become more "magical" or inspired.

1 / First, imagine closing your human, seeing eyes and opening your one, sensing eye. To do this, imagine a blank screen—like a movie screen—behind your seeing eyes, upon which your soul can project images for you to explore and experience on a multidimensional level. Now, project an image of yourself during the happiest time of your life onto that screen—a time in which you were laughing, open, and unafraid.

2 / Then, clear the image from your mental screen and project an image of yourself during the most confident time in your life—a time in which you were glowing, radiant, and empowered. How did you feel in that moment? Can you recall where you were or what you were wearing? Finer details like these help you crystallize your vision during visualization exercises.

3 / Now, clear that image and project an image of yourself today. Where can you love yourself more fully right now, and how can you support yourself more deeply in this moment? What do you need in order to feel happy, loved, and seen? You have activated your Third Eye Chakra now in service of your Highest Good and your needs in this moment.

4 / Imagine the possibilities if you could do the same for others, and for our planet: For instance, if our planet could engage this broader love frequency, perhaps we would see an end to global conflicts. In this way, our Third Eye Chakra becomes a healing tool for all beings: Once we can "see" ourselves clearly, we can "see" others clearly, too. May your vision be of service to you and the entire Collective. And may you and others be healed by what you see with all of your eyes, always.

5 / When you feel connected to your deepest inner knowing and inner channel to the divine, and when you feel that your vision has been fully activated, close your induction with the universal blessing: Amen, A'ho, So it is.

Reflection Questions for the Third Eye Chakra

As you ponder the English name for this chakra—the "third" eye—consider how having another channel for sight could assist you in your life as a healer, as an empath, and then as a sister, a partner, a child, a parent. After all, you possess it in order to be of service to others. As you consider these reflection questions, anoint yourself with an essential oil or perfume blend to activate this additional point of sight. Cypress, mugwort, and blue lotus essential oils are powerful tools to enhance your physical and etheric sight. Diffuse one or all of them, or blend them into a sacred perfume to activate the awareness each tree, herb, and flower offers. You could also drink a tea infused with mugwort and blue lotus to soften your central nervous system and enhance your clairvoyance, or clear sight, as you ponder and respond to the following questions:

1/ Where in your life does your inner vision feel the most accurate? Have you been able to accurately anticipate events and situations before—even if doing so made you uncomfortable or uneasy? If so, what was the outcome?

2/ Where in your life could you use additional insight right now? Imagine a deep indigo light of energy, the sacred Indigo Ray, surrounding your head from the space between your eyes around to the back of your head. See it opening and expanding your ability to see in all directions, before and after you, ahead of and behind you. Give yourself the gift of time to explore what you see. Without judgment, write down key words, phrases, and sentences that describe what comes through.

3/ When you think of yourself as a sacred counselor or visionary, how do you feel? What gifts do you have around sight or vision that could help you or someone you know or love? What gifts of perception or sight do you have that could help someone you have never met, and how can you communicate your vision to those who have no access to it? How will you explain what you see?

When you are ready to close your reflective writing, thank your spirit guides and higher self for attending you while you write, and blow out your candles. Store any gems you've used and other writing tools together in a special place so that you'll have them handy when you want to do more reflective writing in the future.

CORRESPONDENCES FOR THE THIRD EYE CHAKRA

goddesses

PYTHIA, CIRCE, HECATE

rune

LAGUZ

gemstones

AZURITE, BLUE AVENTURINE, LABRADORITE, LAPIS LAZULI, SODALITE, TANZANITE

essential oils/herbs

BETEL LEAF, BLUE LOTUS, CYPRESS, EYEBRIGHT, JUNIPER, MANDRAKE ROOT, MUGWORT, OPOPONAX, POPPY

tarot card

MAJOR ARCANA: THE HIGH PRIESTESS

planet

MOON

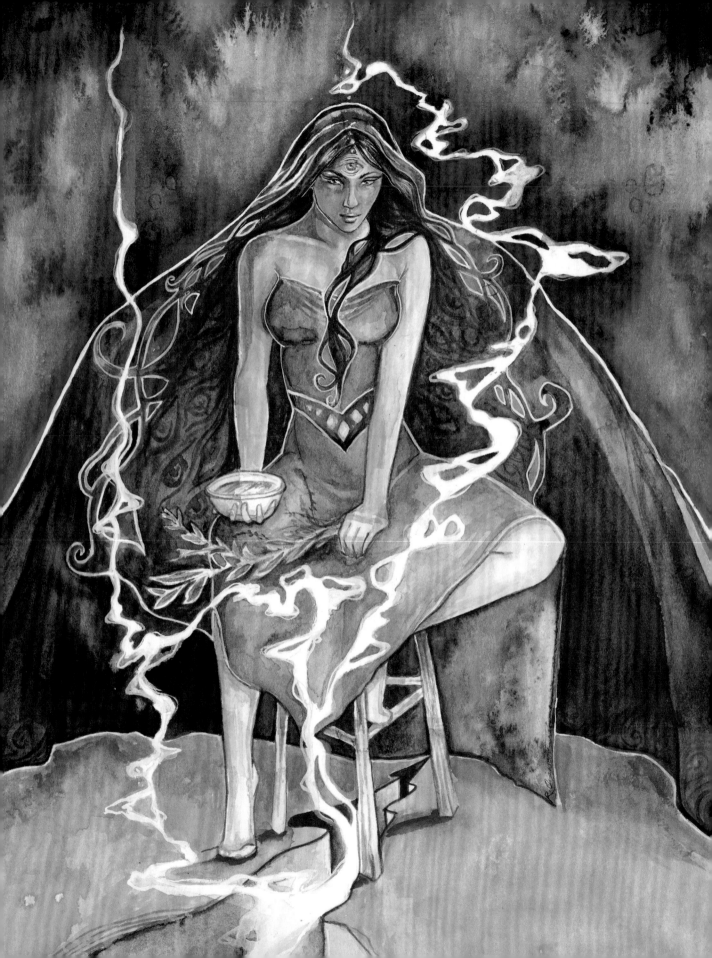

Goddesses of the Third Eye Chakra

Interestingly, in the domain of intuition and the Third Eye Chakra, only three goddesses emerge as our guides on this sacred journey: **Pythia**, **Circe**, and **Hecate**. They are considered goddesses of the threshold, or the doorway between the words of the living and the dead. In many cultures and traditions, healers, *curanderas*, shaman, and other figures of transformational healing are thought to live on the periphery of consciousness and space. From these spaces they see, work, and gaze upon us, but leave us to our own mortal devices to find the cures and mechanisms of healing that align with human modalities and western models of what can cure or "fix" all that ails us.

Pythia is the goddess of the Third Eye, who can connect you to ancestral wisdom, channeled visions, and inner understanding. She is the high priestess of what might be, and is able to sit between the "now" of your current existence and the "then" of what may unfold in the future. Circe is the goddess of magic in the Greek pantheon, but like all goddesses, she carries the magic of light and shadow, love and darkness. She is capable of showing you your own magic—or poisoning your waters, killing all creation. Hecate is the Greek goddess of transformation. She is the goddess of all crossroads: between life and death, between the past and the future, between your goddess self and your human self. The goddesses of intuition show you the many ways you can work with energy, and then it is up to you to find ways to channel their energy productively.

Ask yourself today how you can work more powerfully and intentionally with sight, creation, vision, and manifestation. Seek the companionship of these goddesses who have navigated this complex terrain before you with ease and grace. Seek their counsel with care and diligence, for they have much to teach you. To call upon them, say aloud, "Oracle Goddesses and Goddesses of Third Sight, illuminate me with your wisdom and your visions. I give thanks for your guidance. Amen, A'ho, So it is."

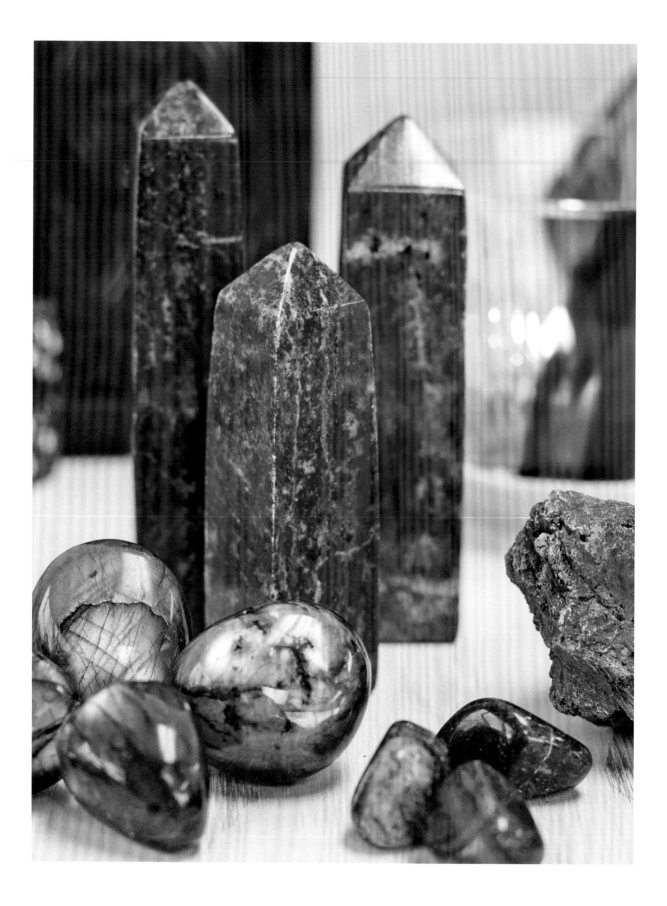

GEMSTONES, ESSENTIAL OILS, AND HERBS OF THE THIRD EYE CHAKRA

Third Eye Chakra Gemstones

AZURITE is the most powerful of all of the Third Eye gemstones, facilitating psychic visions for famed prophets and seers such as Edgar Cayce, who considered it a stone of psychic mastery.

BLUE AVENTURINE heightens intuitive capacity and brings visions of future events, while **TANZANITE** is a healing gem thought to contain teachings in other dimensions. Blue aventurine foretells what will be, while tanzanite reminds you of what has been. Both can be used to improve your experience of the present moment and to guide clients toward their personal Highest Good.

LABRADORITE holds the energy of new possibilities. It contains flashes of rainbow light that ignite the imagination and help you kindle your inner fire. Work with labradorite at the New Moon—or whenever you set intentions for new beginnings—to envision your deepest passions and ignite your inner desires.

LAPIS LAZULI brings confidence and self-esteem to the bearer. In ancient Egypt, it was considered the Queen's Stone of Power. Cleopatra herself quarantined its use and dedicated its power to her own empire-building purposes: She believed it brought her immortality, intuition, and victory.

SODALITE often referred to as the Dreamcatcher Stone, is believed to prevent nightmares and night terrors. It actively helps you release fears of what might be to help you stay present and focused in the moment.

To work with these gems of vision and new beginnings, consider setting up a sacred space or altar for intuition somewhere in your home. This can be done very simply, with just a few crystals and a deep blue or indigo candle.

Placing items on your altar that represent the four elements keeps your sacred space balanced and aligned, which will increase the sense of peace and balance you experience when you spend time there. A chalice of water, an abalone shell, or a vase of fresh flowers invokes the magic of the water element, which enhances intuition and foresight (and adds color and beauty, too). Your chosen gemstones represent the grounding and stabilizing earth element on your altar, while a feather or smudge bundle represents air. The fire element is best represented by a candle in a color aligned to the purpose for the altar.

Once you have your elemental tools in place, begin a routine or practice of sitting before this space for a few minutes each day, saying a brief prayer and calling upon your spirit guides to be with you. If you like, you can beautify the space with an indigo table covering—the color of the Third Eye Chakra—and place your stones in a sacred spiral shape to reflect the energy of intuition, which begins within and then unfolds without.

Enjoy the process of adorning your altar and setting up your sacred space. Add personal touches, such as photographs, if you are called until it feels uniquely and beautifully yours. Then, spend time enjoying them in the moment, without focusing on the past or future. Your altar or sacred space is a gift you give to your soul. May it bless you.

" …**MANDRAKE** ROOT ENHANCES INTUITION IN MATTERS OF LOVE, WHILE **BLUE LOTUS** SOFTENS AND RTVELAXES THE CENTRAL NERVOUS SYSTEM, MAKING IT EASIER TO CONNECT WITH SPIRIT GUIDES.

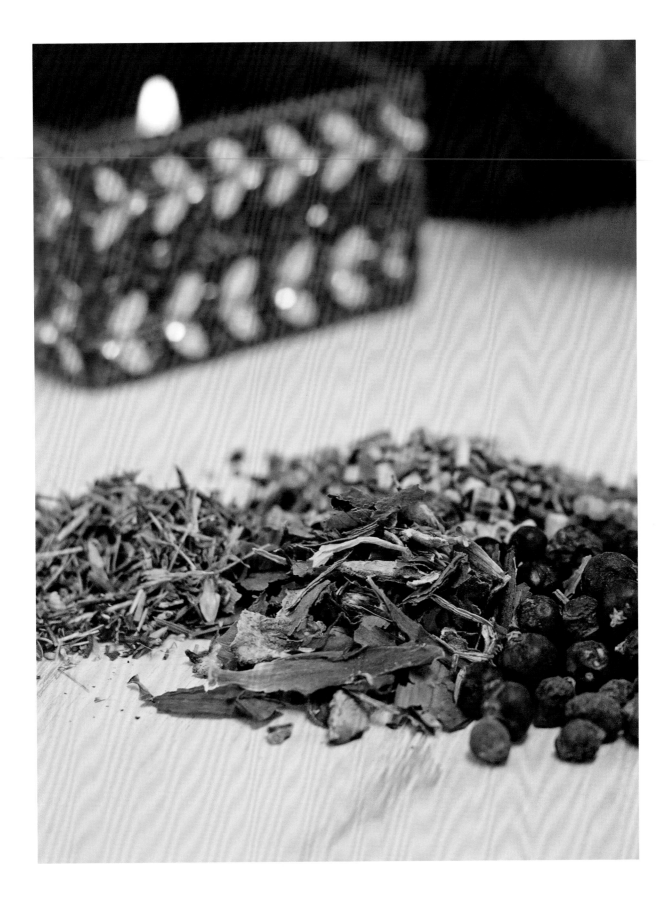

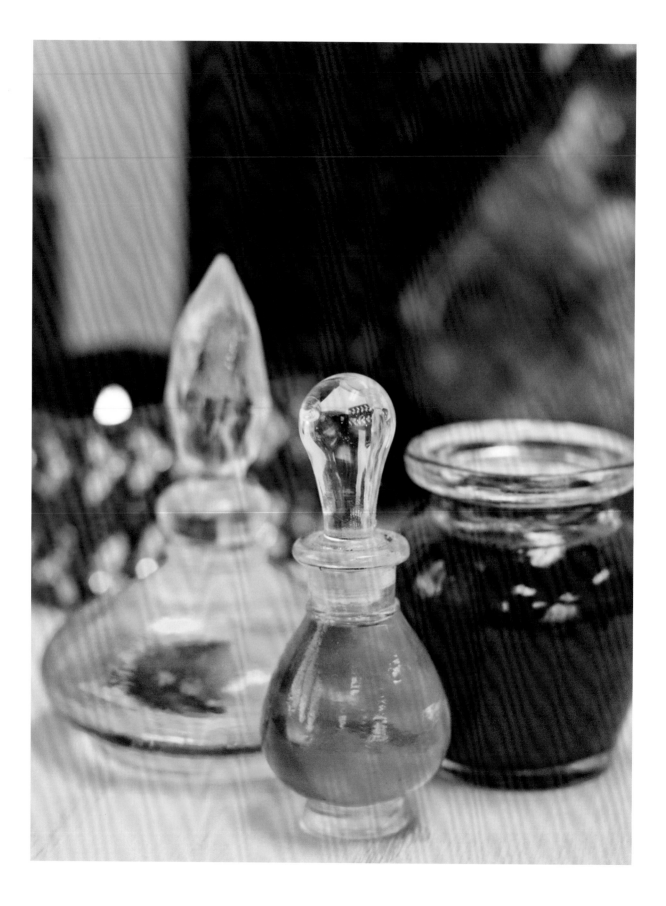

Third Eye Chakra Herbs and Essential Oils

Eyebright brings mental clarity and enhances vision, both human and psychic. **Juniper** offers healing via purification and protection from evil spirits. **Mugwort**, known as the Witch's Herb, has a mild sedative effect and thus has been thought to facilitate deep states of meditation and powerful prophetic visions. **Poppy** calms the mind and prepares you for ceremonial work. **Mandrake Root** enhances intuition in matters of love, while **Blue Lotus** softens and relaxes the central nervous system, making it easier to connect with spirit guides. (Blue lotus was sacred in ancient Egypt and often buried with bodies to ensure safe passage to the afterlife and the soul's final resting place.)

Cypress is considered to be a tree of the dead in many cultures, but in ancient Greece, a ring of Cypress trees circled the famed Oracle at Delphi, and has become known in Greece as a tree of wisdom and intuition. **Opoponax** is an ancient resin that brings protection and transmutation, helping purify and clear stuck or stored energy. **Betel Leaf** has a lengthy history as a sacred plant: It is used in prayer ceremonies and can be burned or used in essential oil form to raise energy frequencies for peace, healing, and intuitive development.

Many of these herbs can be used in various ways to enhance mood and increase psychic awareness. Mugwort and blue lotus, when blended and taken as a tea, help to calm the nerves and open the mind to new possibilities. You can use sprigs of juniper as décor around your home, especially at the holidays, to enhance a deeper level of spiritual engagement and energy.

Hang wreaths made of juniper on the doorway(s) to your home to protect it from intruders. Burn opoponax resin to open sacred space and create an environment suitable for spiritual work and divination. Finally, use the recipe on page 145 to make a powerful Oracle Anointing Blend, which combines the medicines of Third Eye herbs with the gemstones of intuition. Use this blend every time you do a reading for a client or for yourself to open the Third Eye and activate your intuitive gifts.

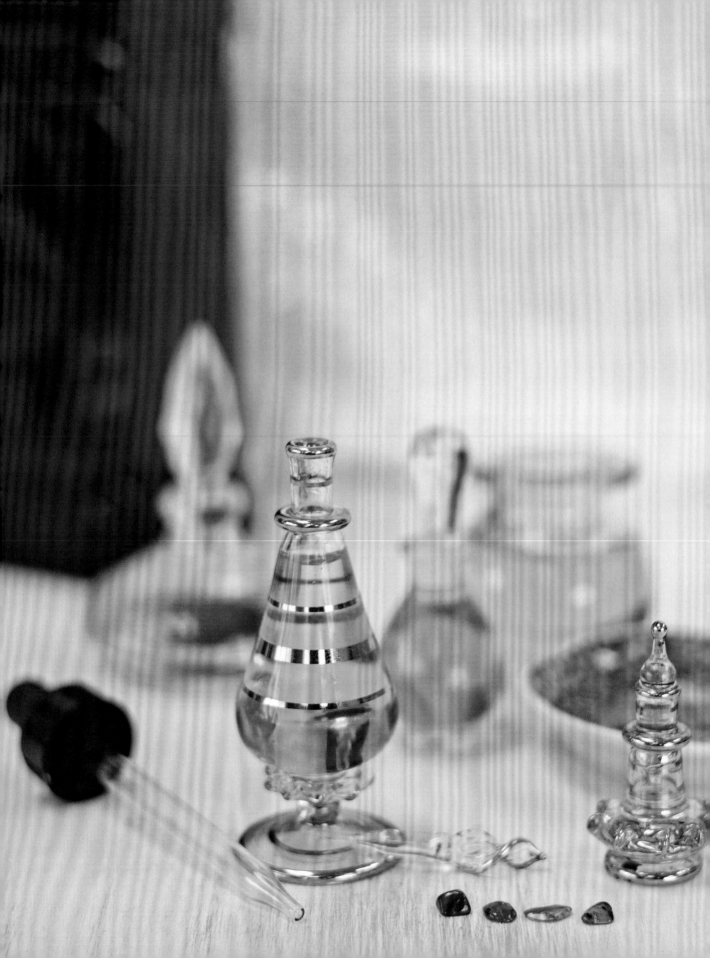

Oracle Anointing Blend

Ingredients

- 10 drops cypress essential oil
- 10 drops blue lotus essential oil
- 5 drops opoponax essential oil
- 5 drops juniper essential oil
- 2 ounces jojoba carrier oil
- 4 chip stones: 1 each of lapis lazuli, tanzanite, blue aventurine, and sodalite

Blend your essential oils together, blessing each oil as you add it to the mixture. Then, place your essential oil blend into a perfume bottle. Fill it to the top with jojoba carrier oil, then add your chip stones. Swirl gently to blend. Set the intention that each time you work with this sacred blend, your intuition will be enhanced and you will see clearly what is needed—for yourself or for your client. Amen, A'ho, So it is.

Tarot Card, Rune, and Planet of the Third Eye Chakra

Major Arcana: The High Priestess

The High Priestess is a figure of mystery and wisdom, and is associated with the Third Eye Chakra. In the Major Arcana of the Tarot, she represents advanced learning and integration of different traditions in service of a comprehensive unifying vision of magic. She honors the sacred texts and prioritizes learning from the past in order to inform her judgment in the present. In this way, she is an open invitation to you to further your own education and improve your understanding of ancient concepts and civilizations, including their traditions and sacred ceremonies. She asks the question: How might you deepen your wisdom in order to connect with the lineages of your ancestral line?

The High Priestess is your most powerful conduit to your past, your present, and your future. Call upon her to access the broader wisdom of your ancestors by asking, "What do I need to know that I do not know today, and how can I integrate that wisdom into the deepest levels of my being?"

Rune: Laguz

Laguz is the rune of the psyche and all that is unseen. As such, it is the primary rune of intuition. Laguz means "lake," and so its watery essence offers the gift of life through wisdom. Water is also the element of prosperity and wealth, so it is also the rune of understanding your personal path to prosperity. This truth will be revealed to you over time as you work with laguz, activating the deepest wisdom once you are ready to receive it. Call upon its energy to help you dive within and excavate the innermost channels of your wisdom. Trust that it is safe to explore your soul's sacred caverns this way.

Planet: Moon

It should come as no surprise that the Moon is the planet of intuition; in so many ways, the moon governs our cycles and our connection to magic. At the New Moon, try to seek wisdom about new ventures, new beginnings, and new possibilities; at the Full Moon, seek gratitude and blessings for intentions that have manifested in the last lunar cycle. Both are occasions for deep connection to intuition and inner wisdom.

Archetypes of the Third Eye Chakra

When you think of intuition, the word "oracle" often comes to mind. Historically, oracles were figures with powers of precognition, who would intuit events before they happened and offer guidance or counsel on the basis of their visions. Thus, the archetype of **The Oracle** presents itself as one face of your own psyche that has unique powers of prophecy and the ability to channel wisdom from outside the self. Like the wise oracles of ancient Greece, the oracle within you is a bringer of wisdom and truth, with a keen ability to envision and foretell the future and to gain clarity and perspective on the past. The Oracle sees all, knows all, and embodies all. She is an open channel of wisdom and understanding that defies human comprehension.

Mantra of the
Third Eye Chakra

In Sanskrit, *Wah yantee* is loosely translated as "wisdom of infinity" and is a mantra you can use to connect to your deepest knowing. The wisdom of infinity knows no beginning or ending; it simply is, and has always been. When you connect to universal wisdom in this way, you are able to let go of anxiety, stress, and fear, since within universal wisdom are energies of peace, alignment, enlightenment, and connection. Recite this mantra when you feel anxious or fearful, which are often signs that you are disconnected from your intuition. When you come back to your deepest wisdom, you will realize that love surrounds you in every way. You are walking the beauty path.

Embodiment Exercise: Third Eye Chakra Activation

When working with any chakra, activation is key. Here, you are activating—or giving permission to—your Seeing Eye to receive and transmit its wisdom via your intuition or inner knowing. Your intuition is your ally in this life, walking the long road of humanity with you as a guide and source of wisdom, truth, and inspiration. All humans are born with innate faith in it, but over time many are taught to trust only facts, science, and what can be seen with their waking eyes. Ironically, many spend the later decades of life trying to return to the state of innocent, open knowing that children so naturally enjoy.

As you develop your intuition, you are by extension engaging your child self, a facet of what Buddhists refer to as the Beginner's Mind, or the ability to meet life with an open mindset. You are silencing the (sometimes very loud) voice of the inner critic and inner skeptic—your adult self—to allow the voice of your inner child and inner oracle to speak from a place of trust and accelerated awareness. Let this meditation guide you.

1/ Close your eyes and imagine yourself as a child, when you were open to new ideas and embraced a freedom of thought that made anything possible. Feel a sense of natural curiosity and warm safety envelop you as you return to that place of trust and understanding. What did you know to be true back then? How can recalling that truth assist you now in trusting the universe to be a safe, welcoming home to your maturing spirit?

2/ Now, imagine a deep indigo—almost violet—ray of light emerging from between your eyebrows. This is the Blue or Indigo Ray of your intuition. Send that beam of light out to the universe and set the intention that it may gather any wisdom, insight, or information you need to access right now in order to live in vibrational harmony with your soul's path. Feel the pulsing indigo beam pushing past our atmosphere, spreading out into the far beyond, gathering information and codes—energy "keys" to unlock health, well-being, peace, or prosperity—for you to use in your life right now.

3/ Ask the beam to collect only information for your highest good that can be used and integrated now (later, if you wish, you can send another beam and ask for long-term guidance or guidance about a specific issue). Say aloud, "Beam of Indigo Light, gather only the wisdom I need to serve my highest good and the highest good of those around me. Amen, A'ho, So it is."

4/ Imagine that Indigo Ray returning to you now, bringing back to you all that you need to know in this moment. Receive the Indigo Ray back at the point of its departure—between your brows. Bless the receipt of the guidance, and give thanks for the gift of wisdom.

May the information you gather bless you, and may the codes you receive heal you. Amen, A'ho, So it is. And on we go.

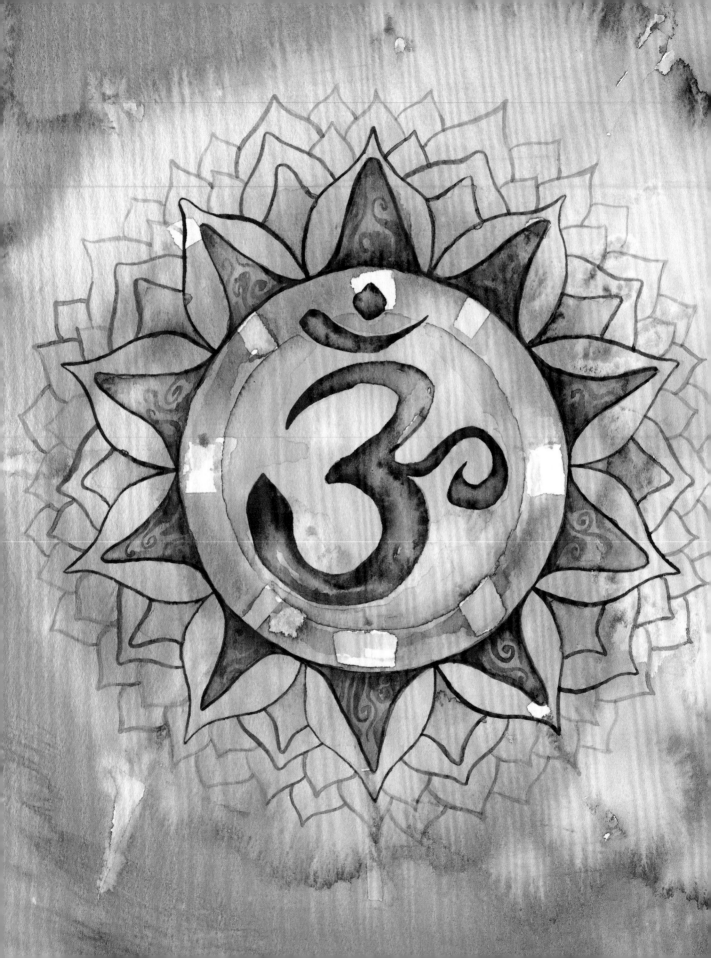

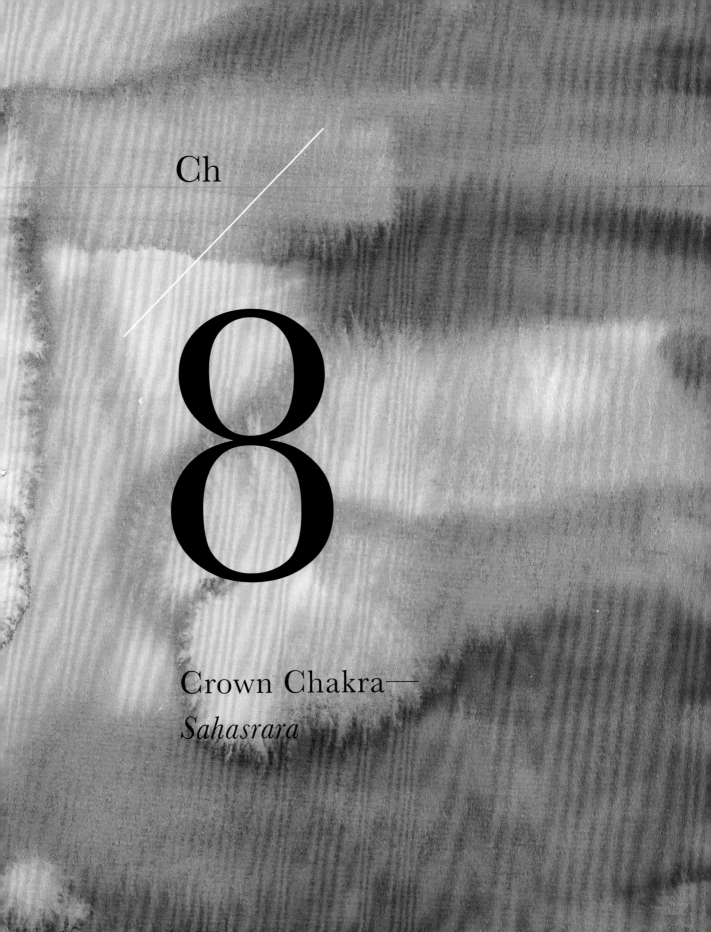

Ch

8

Crown Chakra—
Sahasrara

The Crown Chakra, your crown of holy connection to the Divine, sits at the top of your head, a bright violet disk of light that emanates what we call the Violet Ray of compassionate and protective light. When your Crown Chakra is open and functioning well, you feel intimately aware of your connection to God/Source/Creator energy. When it is blocked or inactive, you feel disconnected from the Divine, and unsure of your relationship to God/Source/Creator.

While most empaths and psychics find it easy to keep an open and clear Crown Chakra through supportive exercises, such as daily meditation and recitation of mantras, many others struggle to find the Divine. It can be difficult to break free of the monotony and routines of everyday life in order to plug into a higher power. And yet we are spiritual beings having a human experience—not the other way around. Thus, the Spirit part of us will always long for a way back to Source.

Anwering the call of your spirit is a powerful gesture. When you say yes to your soul's development, you also say yes to the collective evolution on the entire planet. You are one powerful piece of the broader matrix of energy that surrounds you. Your words, actions, thoughts, and decisions affect everyone around you. The Crown Chakra, your energy sanctuary, is the center of our comprehension of this interconnectedness. When we lose our spiritual way, this is the place we return to remember who we are. Here at the Crown Chakra, you learn that life is not meant to be a constant struggle. There should be flow and ease. You will find both here, waiting for you.

Embodiment Exercise: Crown Chakra Induction

The Crown Chakra is literally your crown of divine wisdom and contact with the divine. Here you are working with the first layer of spirit guides and angelic beings who serve as intermediaries between this realm and theirs. When you want to activate and channel their wisdom, you can use this meditation to guide your exploration of the Crown Chakra and its many inspirational gifts.

1 / Think of the Crown Chakra as a literal crown of amethyst crystals and purple roses, lit from within by the Violet Ray of light. Visualize it glowing above your head, gently resting there. You become an example to others of peace and spiritual awareness just by being, by allowing yourself to receive the energy emitted by this energy center. At the Crown Chakra, we learn the medicine of allowing and becoming.

2 / The Crown Chakra is also a potent source of physical and spiritual healing. While the Heart Chakra is your center of love and compassion, you experience unconditional love at the Crown Chakra, because here you are welcomed, understood, and seen just as you are. Here you are revered and held as a child of all creation. Here you are guided and loved, seen and recognized at the soul level as kindred of the spirit realm. As you open the Crown Chakra, the top of your head may tingle or vibrate, or you may feel lightheaded. These are perfectly natural reactions.

3 / To experience the magic of the Crown Chakra, recognize that within this energy center sits your deepest sovereignty. You are seen here as the queen or goddess, king or god, that you truly are. When you allow yourself to feel your sovereignty—that is, your truly indelible power and divine authority—what feelings arise? Physically, as you connect to your inner power, you might feel dizzy or as if you are floating, or tingling in your hands and feet, as these are other places in the body where excess energies are expelled. These, too, are normal reactions.

4 / When you trust that you are right where you are meant to be in life, in this moment, you access a level of peace few experience. This peace stems from the knowledge that you simply need to be, and, just by being, you change the world. At the Crown Chakra, you are invited to explore your thoughts about yourself and your life, untangling them from old patterns that may have limited you in the past. Rise now to the occasion of your soul and find your power. When you feel ready to receive this freedom, extend your arms out to your sides and allow yourself to feel the flow of energy from root to crown, extended from your feet to the very top of your head and out, side to side, from your left fingertips to your right ones.

5 / Once you feel the surge of energy, which could be experienced as warmth, tingling, coldness, or lightheadedness, relax your arms and bring your attention to the top of your head. Imagine a ring of light surrounding your head, a beacon of truth and wisdom surrounding you now and always. Give thanks for this sacred connection to the Divine and then close this induction with the universal blessing: Amen, A'ho, So it is.

Reflection Questions for the Crown Chakra

Gather a few tools to support you as you consider the meaning of the Crown Chakra as the seat of your spiritual power, sovereignty, and connection to God/Source/Creator energy. Choose a lavender or violet candle, scented with the same essential oils—they are aligned with the Crown Chakra. You might reach for scapolite, a particularly powerful ally. As the stone of success and integration of wisdom, it will assist you as you reflect upon the wisdom of the Crown Chakra. Call in your spirit guides to assist and inspire you as you consider and respond to the following questions:

1 / What is your favorite way to connect with God/Source/ Creator energy right now? When you want to feel more in touch with the Divine, what do you do and where do you go? Is there a person or place who can instantly reconnect you with your sense of divinity? Perhaps there is a piece of music that helps you connect more deeply?

2 / Self-respect is a natural outcome when your Crown Chakra is open, clear, and active. How would you describe your own level of self-respect right now? Where in your life could you enhance your self-respect or encourage others to treat you with more respect? Remember that you are a child of the divine. What does this concept mean to you?

3 / Faith resides at the Crown Chakra as well. Where in your life do you experience profound faith, and where has your faith been tested? When you lose faith, how do you regain it?

When you are ready to close your reflective writing, thank your spirit guides and higher self for attending you while you write, and blow out your candles. Store any gems you've used and other writing tools together in a special place so that you'll have them handy when you want to do more reflective writing in the future.

CORRESPONDENCES FOR THE CROWN CHAKRA

goddesses

SHAKTI, QUAN YIN

gemstones

AMETHYST, AURALITE 23, CHAROITE, LEPIDOLITE, PURPLE FLUORITE, SCAPOLITE, SELENITE, STITCHTITE, SUGILITE, SUPER 7

tarot card

MAJOR ARCANA: THE HERMIT

rune

WUNJO

essential oils/herbs

FRANGIPANI, GOTU KOLA, LAVENDER, PALO SANTO, PINK LOTUS, SPIKENARD, ST.-JOHN'S WORT

planet

JUPITER

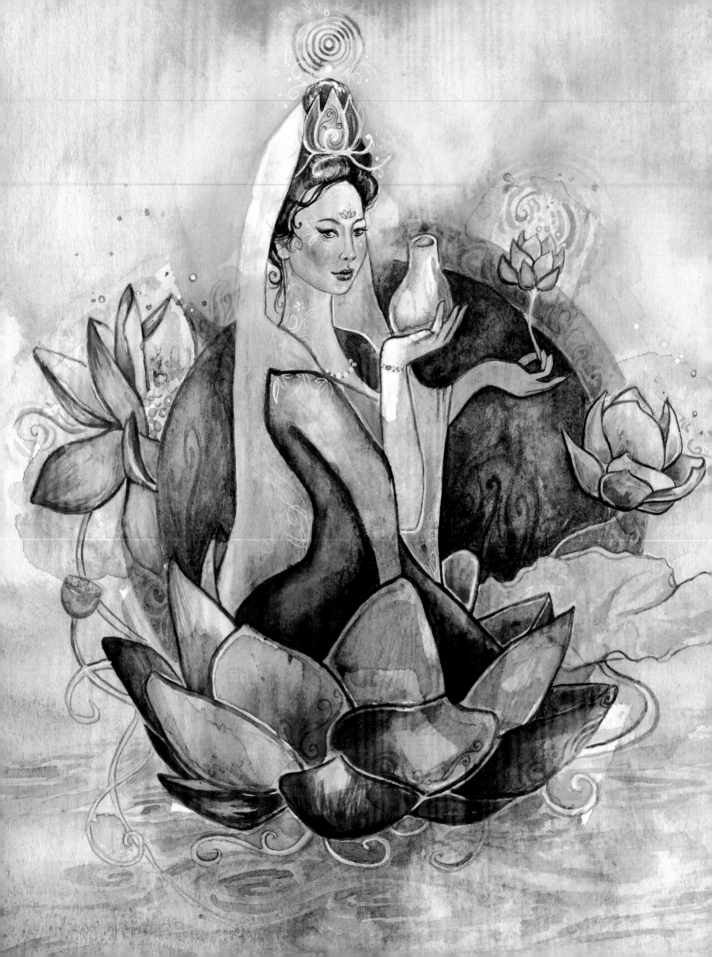

Goddesses of the Crown Chakra

Shakti is the primary goddess teacher at the Crown Chakra, though she is not alone. For example, in the Greek pantheon, Irene is the supreme goddess of peace: You can call upon her to boost your faith and help calm you when you feel anxious or afraid. Shakti, though, embodies all the traits of all the goddesses from every pantheon. She is, in many ways, the most powerful goddess explored in this book. All energies are her energies, and all traditions fall within her domain. In this way, her energy reflects the inclusive energy of this chakra.

The Crown Chakra is your last physical anchor of spiritual energy; after it leaves the Crown, your energy passes out of the range of your physical body. Shakti ensures proper flow of energy from the Third Eye through the Crown and on to the Soul Star Chakra. She filters out any energies that do not serve you and welcomes new energies of peace, serenity, and creative inspiration. When you lose your way, Shakti will guide you back.

Much like the Crown Chakra itself, Shakti offers a higher calling to a deeper level of awareness. As a bridge between the physical and the spiritual, the Crown Chakra supports you as you balance your human and spiritual needs. Call upon Shakti to support you in reconnecting with the Divine Feminine in all its aspects. That means reclaiming your spiritual sovereignty as well as your sexual, creative, emotional, and intellectual sovereignty. After all, the mind and brain are also ruled by the Crown Chakra, and as you think, so you become. Let Shakti guide you as you become your fullest self.

Quan Yin is the secondary goddess of the Crown Chakra, but perhaps an even more central figure than Shakti because she represents embodied compassion. As a *bodhisattva*, or figure of enlightenment, she is the Chinese goddess of divine mercy. Quan Yin uses water to bless and purify, and is often represented as pouring the healing waters of life from her chalice. Her willow branch, another important symbol of her healing capacity, is used to direct healing energies. Keep a chalice of water on your altar to represent Quan Yin's merciful and feminine flow and place a small piece of willow on your altar to represent her ability to direct healing energy toward those most in need. Willow also represents our human capacity to grow, evolve, and become more aligned to the energies of ascended masters like Quan Yin.

Shakti and Quan Yin are both universal figures of creation and compassion who, together, represent the most powerful aspects of Divine Feminine love.

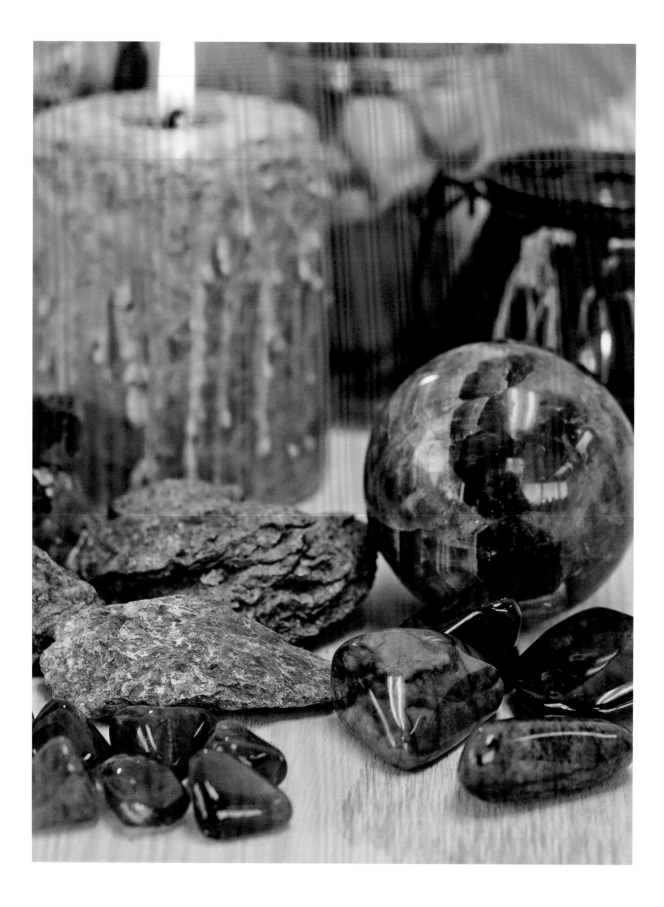

GEMSTONES, ESSENTIAL OILS, AND HERBS OF THE CROWN CHAKRA

Crown Chakra Gemstones

AMETHYST is the most widely accepted gemstone of the Crown Chakra, and for good reason: It purifies, detoxifies, and brings both balance and peace to the bearer.

AURALITE 23 and **SUPER 7** are the master healers of the Crown Chakra gemstones, actively reducing inflammation and helping your body self-heal from emotional and physical trauma.

LEPIDOLITE is micanized lithium, and so it brings powerful peace and relaxation. It relaxes the central nervous column, allowing a flood of soft, flowing energies to move through all energy centers.

PURPLE FLUORITE clarifies your dharma, or soul work, and attracts new opportunities and ways for you to manifest your purpose.

SCAPOLITE is the gemstone of successful outcomes, and helps you organize your thoughts to facilitate clarity.

SELENITE carries a powerful vibration of peace. It clears energy from people, places, and things, but usually does not need to be cleared itself. Thus, it is a powerful ritual tool and can be used to prepare sacred space for ceremonial work.

STITCHTITE promotes the creation and maintenance of strong personal boundaries in relationships, and **CHAROITE**, the Warrior's Stone, offers courage to the bearer.

SUGILITE is a cleanser and detoxifier of the physical body. It raises personal vibration to counteract illness of any kind.

To work with your Crown Chakra gems, consider a form of body gridding called The Crown of Gems. Body gridding is the use of gemstones in physical layouts either on or near the body, and it helps unify the energies of the stones in order to calibrate a person's energies. For example, if you are ill, you might place healing gemstones on or near the afflicted part of the body. By surrounding the top of your head, or Crown Chakra, with Crown Chakra gemstones, you increase the energy frequency of this energy center and facilitate spiritual healing and well-being. Here's how to do this:

1/ Once you are in a comfortable position—preferably lying down without a pillow under your head—place five to ten Crown Chakra gemstones of your choice around the top of your head. Work from left to right, starting at the left ear, plac-ing the stones over the top of your head and continuing all the way to your other ear. (You can use five to ten different stones, or groupings of the same or similar stones, depending on what your intuition calls for.)

2/ Next, imagine the Violet Ray of protective, peace-filled light emanating from the top of your head, connecting all the gems in a band of healing purple light. Feel the heat of the energies as they rise, surrounding your head and bathing it in a warm halo of divine light. Receive the blessings of this light, and remain in this position for as long as your intuition guides you to.

3/ When you are ready, open your eyes, sit up, and gently bring your attention back to present time.

" PINK LOTUS IS CONSIDERED THE SUPREME LOTUS AND BRINGS TRANSFORMATION AND ENLIGHTENMENT.

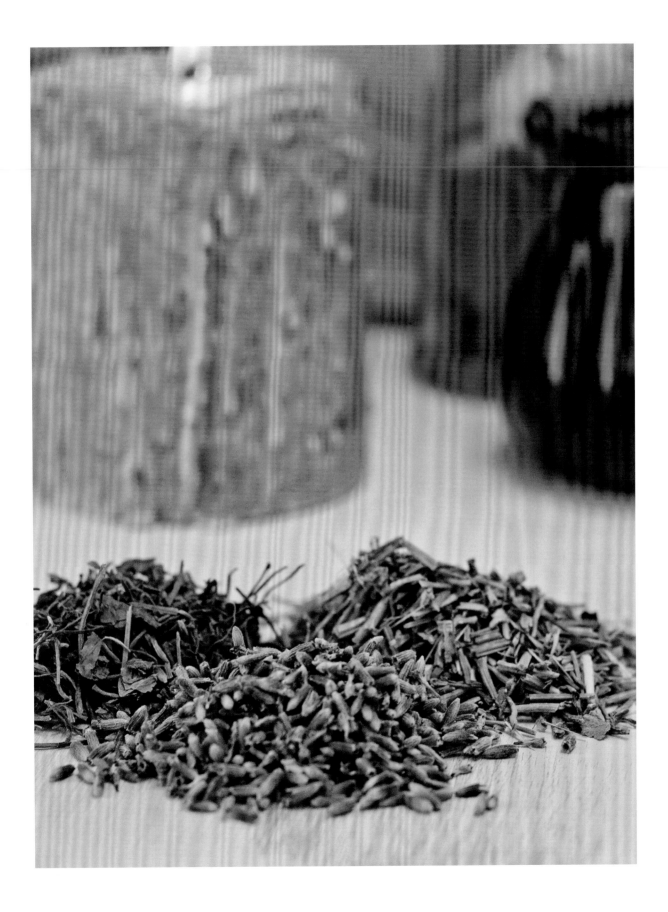

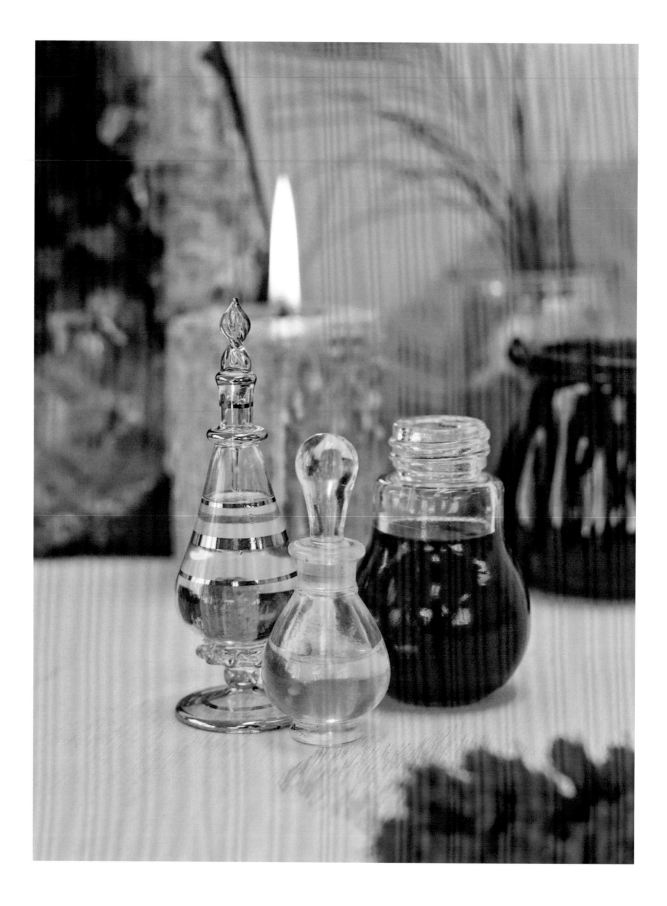

Crown Chakra Herbs and Essential Oils

Gotu Kola deepens your gifts of perception by opening the mind and expanding awareness. Shaman and medicine people in a variety of cultures take it as a preparatory tea or tincture ahead of serious ceremonial work. **Lavender** brings calm and peace and invites a sense of complete well-being when consumed as tea or made into a sweet, fragrant syrup. **Pink Lotus** is considered the Supreme Lotus, and brings transformation and enlightenment. **St.-John's Wort** has long been revered as a treatment for depression and anxiety.

The smoke and essential oil of **Palo Santo** have anti-bacterial and anti-microbial properties, making them ideal tools to fight colds, flu, or illness of any kind. **Spikenard** is the workhorse of the Crown Chakra herbs and essential oils, because it offers so many healing and therapeutic benefits: It has anti-bacterial, anti-microbial, anti-fungal, and anti-aging benefits. Spikenard is also calms the central nervous system, aligns all nine of the chakras, and balances hormones. **Frangipani**, commonly known as plumeria, is a fragrant, magical flower from the South Pacific that thrives in any tropical environment. It attracts universal love and helps you to see that love flows to you from every direction, all the time.

All of the Crown Chakra herbs and essential oils are helpful for relieving anxiety or depression, as each has relaxing and softening properties that are perfect for bringing peace to the overactive or anxious mind. Craft the Peace of Mind Mist (see page 165) and spray it around your space or use it as a light perfume. The addition of an amethyst or lepidolite gemstone to the bottle adds an extra layer of peace magic to this mystical blend!

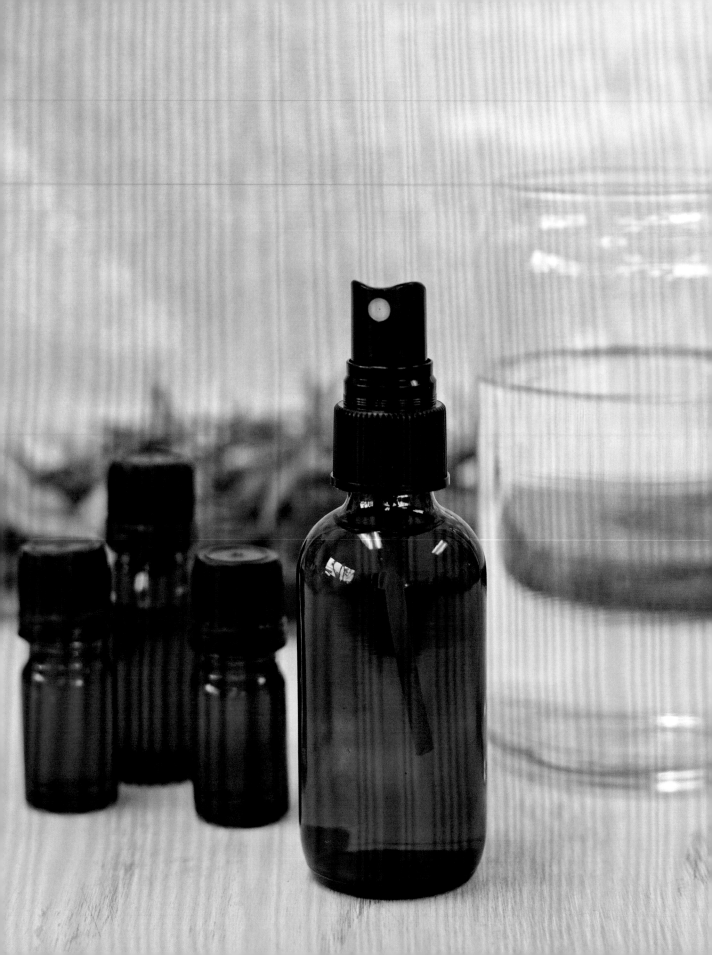

Peace of Mind Mist

Ingredients

- 4 drops lavender essential oil
- 6 drops St.-John's wort essential oil
- 2 drops spikenard essential oil
- 4 ounces (113 g) lavender hydrosol or distilled water
- 1 to 2 lepidolite or amethyst chip stones

First, blend your essential oils, one at a time. As you add each oil to the blend, consider the properties it brings. Next, pour the hydrosol or distilled water into a dark amber or blue glass bottle. (You can choose a bottle with a plastic dropper or a spray cap, but, in general, this blend words best as a spray mist.) Add the essential oils to your hydrosol. Give thanks for the medicine of each essential oil, honoring the spirit of the plant and the gift it is offering you. Then add your chip stones, swirling the mixture with the gems to properly mix the ingredients. Keep this mist near your bed or meditation space, or in any place where you can use more mindfulness and peace energies. Amen, A'ho, So it is.

Tarot Card, Rune, and
Planet of the Crown Chakra

Major Arcana: The Hermit

The Hermit is perhaps the most powerful figure of the Major Arcana, not because he wields direct authority or influence, but precisely because he is a figure with *indirect* authority. His power lies in the lantern he holds, which represents his ability to pave a path of light and beauty in a sometimes-dark world. The Crown Chakra represents this valiant effort to maintain light in dark places, and so The Hermit becomes a figure of validation and inspiration to empaths who do this sacred work every day. It is not easy to be a pioneer, but that is the path of the leader, and the Crown Chakra, in many ways, is the leader of our energy system. It is the launching point for our connection to the Divine. What lies beyond the Crown Chakra is the light of The Hermit's sacred lantern.

To connect with The Hermit's wisdom, ask yourself what your source of light is right now in your life. Where does your illumination come from? And what spaces of the world do you illuminate? Who relies upon you as their source of light and wisdom, and upon whom do you rely for light, support, and direction?

Rune: Wunjo

Wunjo brings happiness and harmony, two of the blessings offered by the Crown Chakra. Wunjo represents the union of the mundane with the spiritual, a point of balance between apparently opposite or competing domains. It is possible to be spiritual *and* grounded; it is possible to live authentically *and* in harmony with others. Wunjo reminds you of the shades of gray that exist in this expansive universe, and the many ways in which binary thinking constrains personal development. To activate the wisdom of Wunjo in your life, ask yourself where you need to experience deeper happiness and harmony in your life. (It might be easier for you to identify places and spaces in your life that are disharmonious; if so, start there.) Allow yourself to answer from a place of transparency and love, and then explore ways you can bring more of whatever you seek into existence.

Planet: Jupiter

Jupiter is the largest planet in our solar system, and it carries powerful energies, too. It represents expansion, growth, possibility, abundance, and trust in a higher power. Jupiter is associated with both Thor and Zeus, the kings of the Norse and Greek pantheons, respectively. Jupiter is the ruling planet of Sagittarius, which is the sun sign associated with freedom through faith. The life lesson of Sagittarius, aligned with Jupiter's meaning, is to trust that a force greater than you has your best interests at heart. While many fear the perceived constraints and prescriptions of organized religion, the true purpose of spirituality is to expand and enhance the experience of life and reinforce the oneness of creation, the connection between and among all living things. Without a connection to each other, it becomes easy to lose faith. If the Crown Chakra is a sacred invitation back to faith and alignment with the rest of the universe, Jupiter is its messenger.

Archetypes of the Crown Chakra

Two primary archetypes guide our understanding and embodiment of the Crown Chakra: **The Channel** and **The Empath**. The Channel is your inner access point to divine wisdom; it is also your highest level of embodiment of Source energy. When The Channel archetype is active, you feel as if you are standing in a wide-open space with easy access to wisdom, insight, and information. Knowledge about your life and your surroundings is easy to access, understand, and interpret, and you feel free from secrets or limitations. Know that The Channel is always an accessible energy stream for you. If you desire more clarity and wisdom, simply call upon this archetype and ask to be shown what it feels and looks like to be the open channel of Source energy. Ask to step into this new reality and feel the liberation of open access to all you need to know.

A related archetype is The Empath. This archetype derives its name from the Greek *empatheia*, or state of emotion, and the ancient Greek root word *pathos*, which means "feeling." The Empath archetype is an archetype of healing, but it is also the archetype of co-dependency in extreme cases: Empaths feel their environments intensely, and must be careful not to entangle their experiences with those of clients. Both of these archetypes, The Channel and The Empath, should use their gifts with care, and be mindful of their energy environments. Techniques for shielding and bubbling up the aura can be very helpful for these particular archetypes: See the Bubble and Zipper Meditations on pages 169 and 170.

Mantra of the
Crown Chakra

There is a difference between the literal meaning of the Sanskrit mantra *Om Namah Shivaya*—"I bow to Shiva"— and its figurative meaning, which is so potent it almost defies description. Names of deities are believed to carry their energy and essence, and Shiva, of course, is one of the most powerful deities of any civilization across history. One of the three deities in the Great Trinity of the Hindu tradition, Shiva is both creator and destroyer. So when you wish to speak something into creation, ask for what you seek and then seal your intention with the mantra *Om Namah Shivaya*. Having done so, you will seal your intention with a blessing capable of moving major obstacles and facilitating a vibrational flow that can manifest thoughts in physical form. Words are powerful, and Shiva is our reminder that as you speak, so events unfold. Mind your words, and use them with care. Each can be a blessing.

Embodiment Exercise:
Bubble and Zipper Meditations

The meditation exercises that follow are very helpful if you feel that your energy is too open and others have too much access to your energy field. (Signs of energy overwhelm, which signal open access to your energy field, are physical and mental fatigue, irritability, confusion, exasperation, and loss of interest in spiritual activities. The Bubble Meditation below helps you encase your energy field in a bubble of light that is impenetrable to outside influence without your permission, while the Zipper Meditation on page 170 offers you a chance to mindfully seal off access to your energy reserves in cases where you feel your boundaries are being violated. Use both, or whichever one resonates most powerfully with you.

The Bubble Meditation

1 / Relax your body and bring your attention to your breath, which will naturally bring you into present time. Next, become aware of your body's comfort level. Make any adjustments needed so you can be fully here, now.

2 / Imagine a huge bubble of translucent white golden light in front of you, about a foot (30 cm) taller and wider than you are on all sides. See this bubble of light gently float on the Earth before you, vibrating and glowing from its center outward. You may even feel warmth as you envision it. Take a step forward, reach out your hand, and touch the sphere of light. Notice how it vibrates back to you, easily and openly inviting contact.

3 / Take another step forward, and see yourself step inside this sphere of light. See the energy move out and open to accommodate you and then close and gently seal itself behind you, enveloping you. Notice how the cares of the world fall away: Here you are safe; here you are well; here you are whole.

Here you are held by spirit guides and are in the care of guardian angels. Here there is no need for anxiety, as time does not exist inside the bubble of light. There is only this moment, which is safe, beautiful, and open to you. Release your concerns about yesterday or tomorrow, and let your body relax and soften. All that matters is right here, right now. Know that all is unfolding in perfect time and order. You only need to be and allow. Give thanks for the protection that surrounds you in this bubble of divine and holy light.

4 / When you are ready, you can choose to emerge and return to your waking state of conscious awareness. Take with you the peace that was gifted to you here, and find ways to mirror it in your daily conversations and actions. Embody the peace you now know exists and is always present, waiting for your acknowledgement.

Amen, A'ho, So it is.

The Zipper Meditation

1/ Relax your body and bring your full attention to this moment, to your breath, and to the feeling in your physical body. Imagine that all of your energy centers are open, and feel each one, from Earth Star to Crown, vibrating and connecting you to the energy it represents. At the Earth Star Chakra, you are completely connected to your ancestors and to the plants and mineral spirits of the underground realms. At the Root Chakra, your roots connect to the Earth itself and you feel yourself safely grounded in the present moment, aware of and grateful for all that surrounds you.

2/ Next, allow yourself to explore and indulge your deepest sensual and creative fantasies at the Sacral Chakra. Then open the Solar Plexus Chakra to experience your most profound sense of personal power. Afterward, the Heart Chakra opens to you, connecting you with love energies and energies of sweet compassion that represent your feminine softness. The Throat Chakra opens next, helping you see and embody your deepest truth. Then the Third Eye Chakra displays all the visions needed to guide and support you from a place of deep knowing and intuition.

3/ Return to the Crown Chakra, and with your hands folded over your heart space, give thanks to Great Spirit for your connection to Source. Having come full circle, honor, acknowledge, and give thanks to the energies that have opened and made themselves available to you.

4/ Then, beginning at the Earth Star Chakra, imagine a giant zipper sitting at the base of all of your energy centers. This zipper will help you close and seal all of your sacred chakras, one at a time, rendering them inaccessible to anyone but you. (This exercise will protect you during times of fear or anxiety.) Pull the zipper northward from your Earth Star Chakra, over the Root, Sacral, and Solar Plexus. Continue over your Heart, Throat, Third Eye, and up to the Crown. Finally, pull the zipper up to the top of your Soul Star Chakra (see page 172).

5/ Close the zipper tightly and feel it seal safely, covering any holes or spaces in your energy field. Know that you are held and safe here, and that nothing can enter your energy field without your permission.

6/ When you are ready to unzip the chakra system—and you should be sure to do so if you wish to begin energy work of any kind, as the flow of energies is critical for creation— release them one at a time, unzipping slowly until all chakras are exposed. You can still keep the chakras protected even if the system itself is unzipped: To engage this layer of protection, simply imagine the entire chakra column encased in a bubble of divine white light of love and peace. This is an additional step and layer of protection for times of need.

7/ Once you feel that your energy centers are protected to your satisfaction, give thanks to your spirit guides for their presence and then release them. Know that you can repeat this exercise any time you feel you need additional energy protection or buffering.

Amen, A'ho, So it is.

Embodiment Exercise:
Crown Chakra Activation

Now that you have explored your crown of power and peace, you have a deeper sense of what it means to commune and connect with your spirit guides. Peace begins the moment in which you realize you are not divided from the Divine. To bring this peace and divine connection into daily life requires a disciplined practice and commitment to living from a place of inspired purpose. Here at the Crown Chakra is where people find the meaning that has seemingly eluded them for a lifetime—even though it has been here all along.

1/ First, stretch your arms out to your sides as far as you can, and take a deep cleansing breath, filling your diaphragm and bathing your cells with your life force.

2/ Envision a violet beam of light, the Violet Ray of peace and protection, glowing brightly and emanating from the top of your head. See it flowing and feel its gentle glow blessing you and your entire auric field as it spreads and grows stronger.

3/ Now, imagine that beam of light becoming a liquid fountain of violet light, flowing and spreading out in front of you and behind you, to the four corners of the Earth and beyond. As each drop of liquid light touches objects around you, see them changed and transformed from within, glowing in a new way with this infusion of life force and spirit force energies.

4/ Spread this healing light wherever you feel called, to the people and places who need it most around the world. You might even think globally, to countries and continents that could benefit from this healing energy stream. Let it flow freely with no expectation that it—or any reward—will return to you.

5/ Now, receive this light of divine love and peace for yourself. Call it in, let it flow over and through you, above and below you. Give thanks for the way in which it already knows where to flow and how, touching each part of you that needs its sacred blessings.

6/ Ask this light to illuminate your spiritual path and guide you to the places and experiences that will inspire, support, and nourish you. Ask it to bathe you in a light that others will recognize, and commit now to living in alignment with that light.

May this peace and purpose illuminate your soul forever. Amen, A'ho, So it is. And on we go.

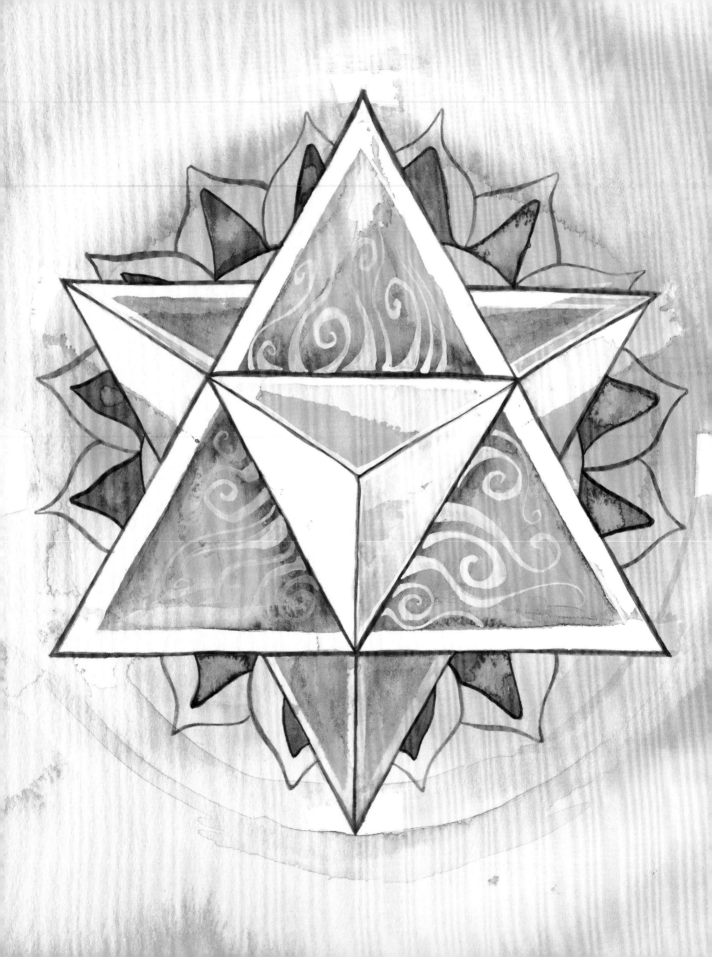

Ch

9

Soul Star Chakra—
Sutara

The ninth chakra is our connection to the stars. It is our portal or access point to other dimensions and provides us with encouragement to pursue ascension and spiritual development in this life. For some, the call of the Soul Star Chakra is louder and harder to ignore; for others, the call is subtler. Whichever way this chakra speaks to you, you can draw from this well of soul strength for inspiration and courage.

The Soul Star Chakra sits about 12 inches (30 cm) above the top of your head and is your aura's uppermost point of contact with the broader energy field. Its alternate name, *Sutara*, means "holy star" in Sanskrit and reflects the sacred nature of the etheric energies that reside beyond the physical chakra system. When this chakra is open and energy is flowing well through it, you feel a sense of embodied peace. You feel capable of channeling and holding the energies around you and find that your manifestation abilities are strong. At the Soul Star Chakra, it becomes possible to imagine a highly complex universe in which time and space are not linear, and where it is possible to experience the past, present, and future synchronously. Consider what it would mean for you, personally, to be able to experience the past now, in this moment, as if it were happening right now. What about the future? What would it mean for you to experience the future now, synchronously with the present? Would you live differently or love differently? And would this wisdom help you or hurt you?

Once your horizons expand and your awareness opens, it is difficult to return to ignorance. The Soul Star Chakra offers you enhanced awareness, but will you be able to integrate it and use it wisely in service of your highest good?

Embodiment Exercise:
Soul Star Chakra Induction

If the Crown Chakra is your crown, the Soul Star Chakra is your halo. It is an angelic amulet, a divine ray of heavenly light that offers nothing but pure nourishment and loving balm to your soul. The medicine of the Soul Star Chakra is ascension, and its call is to the deepest part of your soul. Use this meditation to guide you on your journey.

1/ If you are ready to answer the call of the Soul Star Chakra, stretch your arms above your head, directly up toward the sky, and point your fingertips skyward. Now, imagine the tips of your fingers making contact with the warmest, most tender energy you have every experienced. It is as if a cloud of love is being placed upon your fingertips.

2/ Pull this radiant energy toward you and hold it gently in your fingers, resting it on the palms of your hands. Imagine it as a luminous soap bubble—delicate and perishable, yet real and palpable. Some say the Soul Star has a six-pointed star of energy within it. Lift your head to gaze into this energy, and see the rays of the star radiating toward you. Each of the six rays carries a message for you: The first ray brings you love; the second, prosperity; the third, peace; the fourth, wisdom; the fifth, beauty; and the sixth, sovereignty. These are the six gifts of Spirit.

3/ Receive each of these blessings as you hear the angel guides and ascended masters who reside here speaking to you. They are saying: May you know love; may you experience prosperity; may you live in peace; may you receive wisdom; may you walk in beauty; may you enjoy sovereignty. (While many receive spirit gifts at the Crown Chakra, you might also notice an opening of your heart space. Be open to receiving the resonance of these gifts wherever they arrive.)

4/ Give thanks for these gifts, and commit to bearing the responsibilities they bring. For you are a teacher, a guide, a leader, and a healer. To conclude this meditation, ask yourself how you can bring these gifts forward in the world, and ask your spirit guides for the strength to do this sacred work with power and reverence. Amen, A'ho, So it is.

Reflection Questions for
the Soul Star Chakra

The Star has been a sacred symbol throughout time, representing human form and spirit connection, and the Soul Star, or Holy Star, is the place within where the human self and star self unite. In Cherokee legends, humans descend from the Pleiadians, a fifth-dimension civilization living in an adjacent star system. These beings are said to live in love and peace, free from conflict. What it would mean for you to love this way, absent from conflict or challenge?

Pour yourself a glass of hydrating spring water, and place a piece of clear quartz inside the glass to raise the frequency as you drink. Imagine that every molecule of the water heals every cell in your body. Receive the healing, allowing yourself to experience the increased frequency, and enjoy the vibration of pure love as you consider the answers to the following questions:

1 / What is becoming clear to you about people and things in your life as you sip this enhanced water? In this place of pure divine love, you are gaining a deeper sense of clarity than ever before. Use this clarity to examine your relationships: Where can you love more deeply or bring more compassion to others in your life now?

2 / Expanding consciousness means you become more aware of subtle energy patterns around you. What methods have you used to integrate your deepening awareness? For example, are you more aware of changes in your sleep patterns or menstrual cycles? Are you more attuned to the rhythms of nature, or have you become more deeply attuned to your own intuition?

3 / How can you celebrate your own personal and spiritual evolution? Your soul is evolving and you are moving closer to your purpose for being. What can you do today to acknowledge this achievement? For instance, you might create an intention space in your home or garden—a corner of your world where you can gather sacred items such as candles, gemstones, essential oils, sea shells, sand, dried flowers, or any talismans that represent your development. Create this space on a day of meaning, such as the anniversary of a significant event. Then tend the space with care either daily or weekly, adding or removing items as they become more or less relevant to you. By celebrating your progress, you ensure its continuation.

When you are ready to close your reflective writing, thank your spirit guides and higher self for attending you while you write, and blow out your candles. Store any gems you've used and other writing tools together in a special place so that you'll have them handy when you want to do more reflective writing in the future.

CORRESPONDENCES FOR THE SOUL STAR CHAKRA

goddesses

WHITE BUFFALO CALF WOMAN, ASHERASH, MOTHER MARY

gemstones

DANBURITE, DIAMOND, HERDERITE, HERKIMER DIAMOND, MOLDAVITE, OPTICAL CALCITE, RAINBOW MOONSTONE, SCOLECITE

tarot cards

MAJOR ARCANA: TEMPERANCE AND THE STAR

runes

DAGAZ, EIHWAZ

essential oils/herbs

ANISE, BASIL, DAVANA, ELEMI, GARDENIA, RED MYRTLE, TUBEROSE, WHITE LOTUS

planets

NORTH AND SOUTH LUNAR NODES

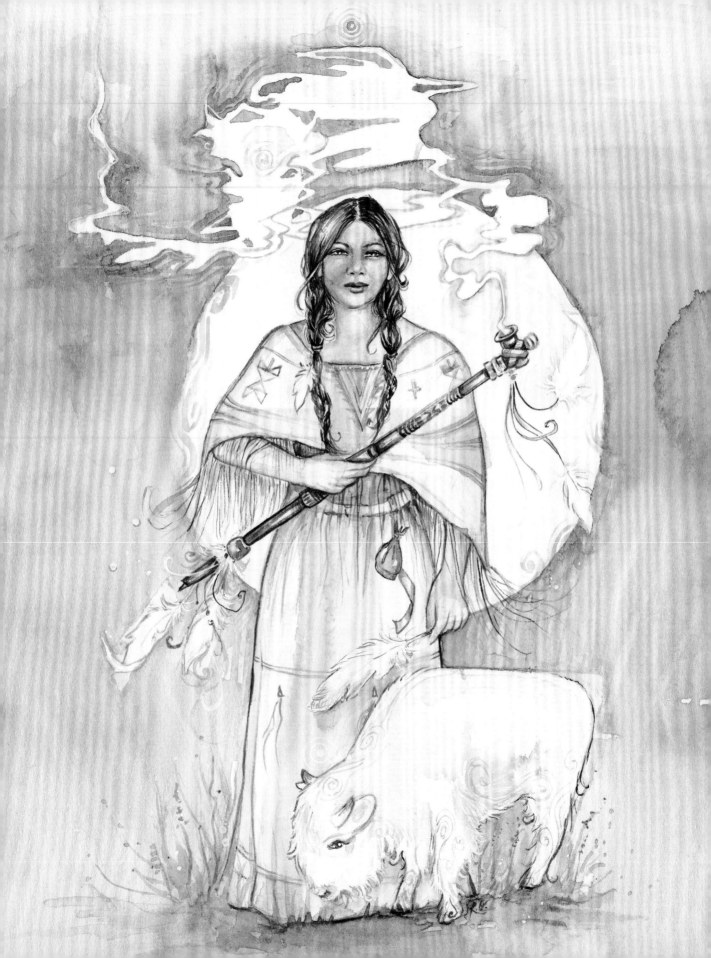

Goddesses of the
Soul Star Chakra

White Buffalo Calf Woman, from the Lakota tradition, is one of several goddesses aligned with the Soul Star Chakra; **Asherah**, the Queen of Heaven in the Semitic and Akkadian traditions, and **Mother Mary** from the Christian tradition, are also associated with the Soul Star Chakra. All three reflect the most heavenly embodiments of Soul Star Chakra energy, which some refer to as Christ Consciousness: the purest essence of divine love manifested on Earth in human form. All of the deities associated with this chakra are teachers: They are ascended masters and light beings who stand between the worlds of the living and the ascended in order to transmit wisdom, love, and light.

White Buffalo Calf Woman was the most influential figure in Lakota lore. She is revered as a mystical figure who taught the Lakota methods for ensuring their well-being and helped them manifest an abundance of resources. Buffalo is sacred to the Lakota, and it is said that the White Buffalo Calf Woman appeared to them one night after a period of drought and famine. She taught them sacred ways of praying and holding space, and promised that if the Lakota would follow her ways, they would never go hungry again. So it was that the Lakota enjoyed an abundance of buffalo, and they developed ceremonial practices that brought peace to the people and the land. Even today, the sight of a rare white buffalo is considered a sign from White Buffalo Calf Woman that you are safe and blessed.

To connect with these queens of heaven, compassion, love, and ceremony, imagine yourself shapeshifting into a white dove. Watch yourself fly and float up to the heavens effortlessly, weightlessly carried on the winds. In this state of effortless peace, give thanks to these goddesses for their blessings of ascension and Christ consciousness.

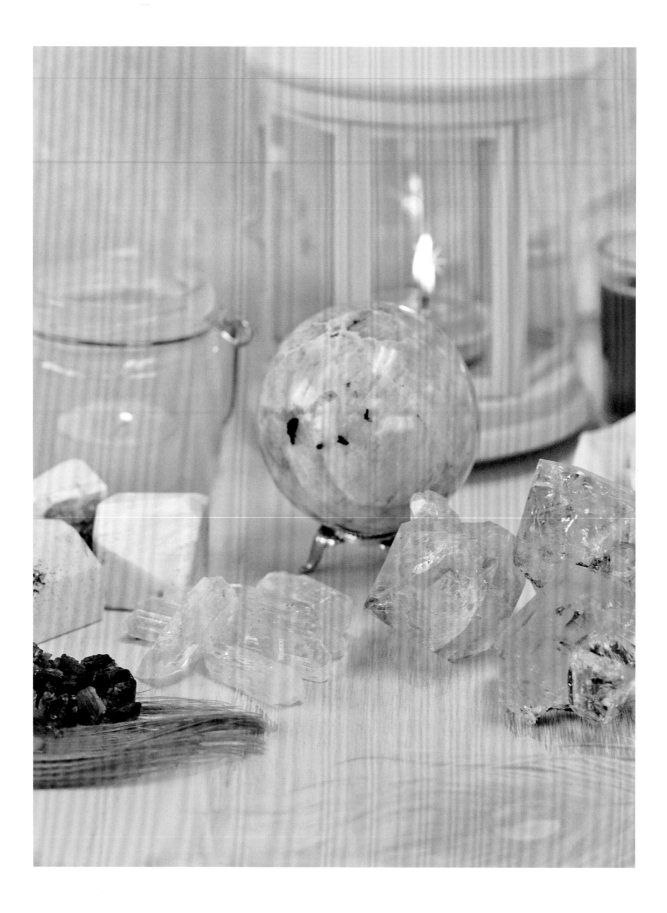

GEMSTONES, ESSENTIAL OILS, AND HERBS OF THE SOUL STAR CHAKRA

Soul Star Chakra Gemstones

Natural **DIAMOND** is the hardest gemstone on the planet. It is formed from carbon, which, metaphysically, is the substance known to be the basis of creation and healing. Diamond reminds you of your inner strength and offers endurance, tenacity, and pure vibration of unconditional love. It is considered to be the most powerful gemstone talisman you can use for channeling the strength of the life force.

DANBURITE is a healer, helping you identify and remove the root causes of pain and discomfort in the physical body. Place danburite on the physical body and wait for tingling or warmth on the skin, which can be a sign that physical healing is needed.

HERDERITE, also a member of the Synergy 12, enhances intuition and expands consciousness. Of all the Soul Star Chakra gemstones, herderite is the most powerful for accelerating spiritual development. Add it to your manifestation altar to help expedite your manifestation and creation efforts.

HERKIMER DIAMOND is said to be the highest vibrational crystal on the planet, and it is collected by gem lovers because of its rarity and clarity. Place a Herkimer diamond above your head during meditation to connect to your Higher Self, a source of powerful wisdom and clarity that can help you identify and evolve into your soul's highest calling.

MOLDAVITE is deep translucent green meteoric glass, the result of a collision between meteors and Earth over Germany, the Czech Republic, and Moldova. (It has never been found or sourced from any other locations.) It is said to hold the energy of the outer edges of our universe and can transfer information from other dimensions and star systems to the person working with it.

OPTICAL CALCITE is an interdimensional travel stone that also brings clarity. Gaze into a piece of optical calcite to see a situation or energy pattern with new clarity and enhanced perspective.

RAINBOW MOONSTONE is the gem of fullness and fruition and carries a joyful energy of celebration, gratitude, magic, and possibility. It can be used in water or charged under full moonlight to create a potent energy elixir of joy and manifestation.

SCOLECITE is the ascension stone. It is a member of the rare Synergy 12 configuration of gemstones and minerals, a category of gemstones said to accelerate human development and manifestation abilities. Carry or meditate with scolecite to connect to universal consciousness and higher dimensional states of awareness.

If you don't have a dedicated meditation space in your home yet, consider this chapter an invitation to create one, and use the energy of the Soul Star Chakra gemstones to raise the most pure, perfect vibrations in your sacred space. This space should be peaceful, silent, and beautiful. Gather the Soul Star Chakra gemstones that speak to you, and decorate your space with those stones and white or cream-colored fabrics, as white is the color of the Soul Star Chakra. Hang twinkling lights to bring a bit of glamour and magic to your space in the evening, or use candles or tealights to add a spark of fire element energy to this peaceful oasis. Light a white candle each time you sit before this sacred space, and anoint yourself with white floral essential oils that resonate with you (see page 187).

" **BASIL** ATTRACTS PROSPERITY, AS DOES **RED MYRTLE**, AND BOTH ARE HELPFUL FOR MEDITATION AND RELAXATION.

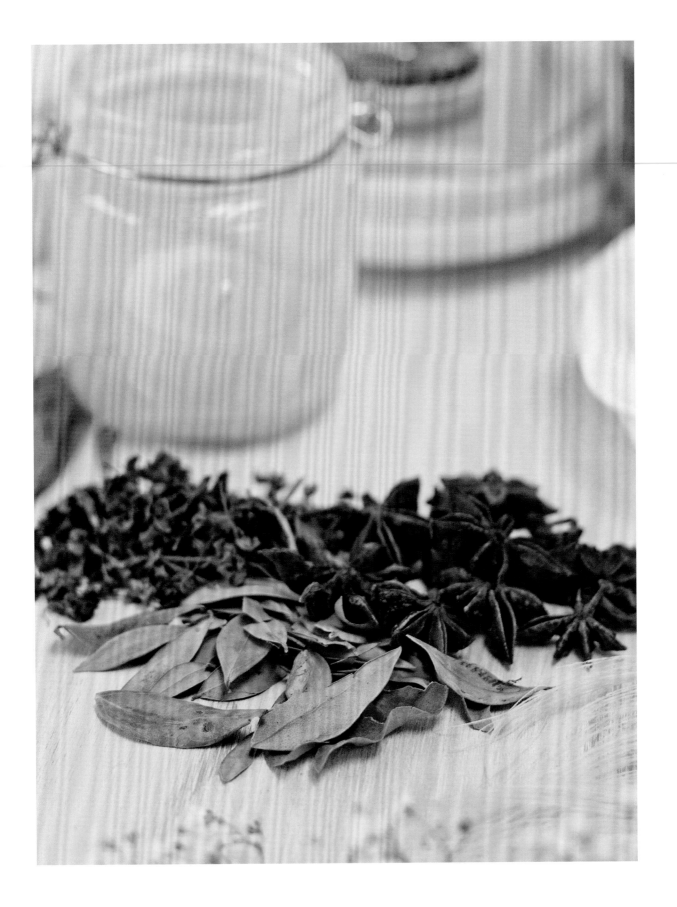

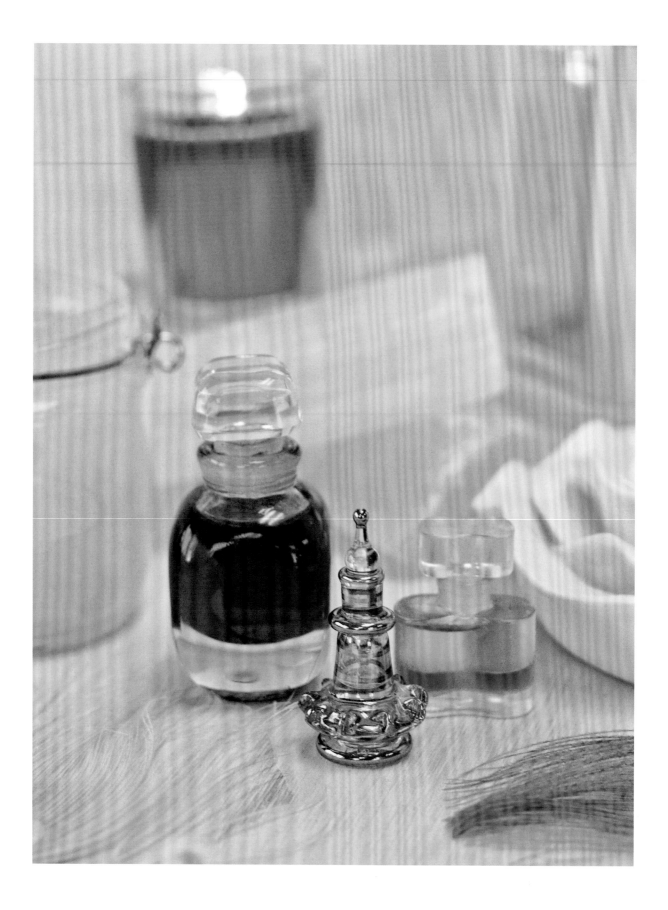

Soul Star Chakra Herbs and Essential Oils

The herbs and essential oils of the Soul Star Chakra are bringers of light. They have angelic energies to them, although each manifests those energies in different ways. **White Lotus** is the womb of creation, connecting you with energies of rebirth. **Anise** makes it easier to hear the voice of your intuition. It is also considered a sacred offering to Source or Great Spirit, especially in its perfect star form. **Basil** attracts prosperity, as does **Red Myrtle**, and both are helpful for meditation and relaxation. **Davana** is useful for divination and psychic visions, and for awakening intuitive abilities and recalling past life memories. **Gardenia** is a spiritual healer, and offers relief to those who have suffered spiritual or psychological trauma. **Elemi** was once used in ancient Egypt during burial and mummification ceremonies, so it is no surprise that it supports transition, new beginnings, and internal transformation. **Tuberose** calms and soothes, promoting relaxation and surrender while easing sadness and anxiety.

A beautiful, comforting way to connect with the energy of the Soul Star Chakra is through a ritual cleansing bath. By using salt, flowers, essential oils, and dried herbs to smudge and purify your space, you can transform the energies around you and within you, opening and preparing you for meditation or ritual work. Plus, ritual bathing has been part of magical preparation processes since ancient times, for the water is a symbol of ritual purification, especially when salt is added. Gather the gemstones, essential oils, candles, plants and flowers, plus any other tools you feel called to include, and begin building a bath altar to bless your watery oasis with peaceful Soul Star Chakra energy (see page 187). Consider including a sacred chalice filled with your favorite beverage, or a vintage glass vase holding fresh flowers aligned to the chakra, such as white roses or peonies.

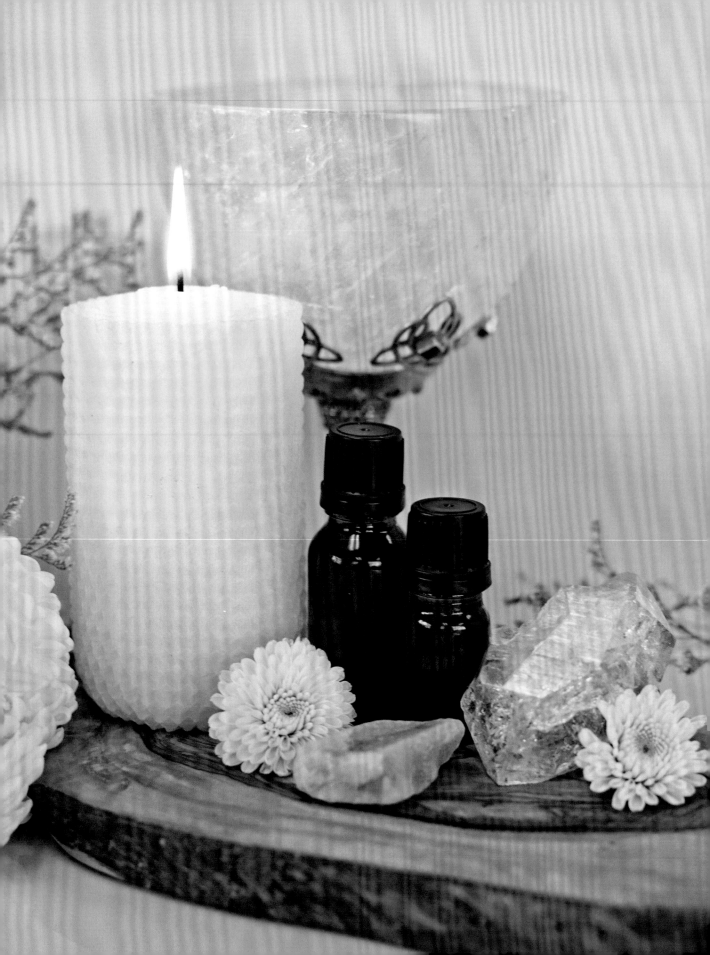

Soul Star Ritual
Bath Altar

Ingredients

- White candle

- Soul Star gemstones

- Soul Star essential oils, such as white lotus, gardenia, and tuberose

- About 2 ounces (57 g) Dead Sea salt crystals

- Fresh roses or other flowers you love

- A sacred beverage to enjoy during your bath, served in a beautiful chalice or stemmed glass

Gather these tools and place them around your bathtub in a clockwise direction, pausing to pray over each item and invoke its energies as you enjoy your ritual bath. Light your white candle, and call upon the Star People to bless you with wisdom and clarity as well as the peace of divine love and connection. Allow yourself to visualize the Six Rays of Soul Star Chakra blessings; receive those blessings now. Run hot water in the bath, and gather the salt in your hands. Pour a few drops of the essential oils over the salts in your hands, then blend them between your fingers, whispering prayers and blessings as you do so. You can even blow your breath on the salts to offer your life force energies to the spirits that will attend you during this ritual bathing experience.

As you take a step into the bath, feel the warmth of the water envelop you. Surrender to its delicate power, letting it cleanse you of any energies that no longer serve you. Set those energies free upon the tiny waves of water you create by running your fingers through the bath gently, side to side. Let your vision go soft and blurry, enjoying the moment and releasing everything else.

Give thanks for this ability to let go and let God. You are a child of the divine, a blessed creation of Source/God/Creator. Stand tall in this identity and allow its power to fuel you from a place of love and service. In this way, you ascend to a higher level of dimensional awareness, and you free yourself from limitations imposed upon you by external forces and pressures. Give thanks for the blessings that surround you, as well as for your ability to see and receive them. Amen, A'ho, So it is.

Tarot Cards, Runes, and Planets of the Soul Star Chakra

Major Arcana: Temperance and The Star

In the Major Arcana of the Tarot, two cards are aligned with the Soul Star Chakra: Temperance and The Star. Temperance represents the ultimate balance and union of forces. The dual chalices often depicted on the front of this card are visual metaphors for the two worlds balanced by humans: the spiritual and the mundane. Back and forth the waters flow in our lives, anchoring in the material realm and then uplifting in the spiritual realm. The Star card offers you the blessing of a wish come true: Before making this wish, give thanks to The Star for reminding you that hope is always available to those who seek it. Let her blessings of wishes come true remind you to believe in magic.

To connect with these two cards, ask yourself where the spiritual energies and mundane energies of your life manifest and co-exist within you. What spiritual qualities or experiences are you seeking to manifest right now, and what support do you need in doing so? What about the mundane or material qualities you are seeking to manifest? Articulating your needs and intentions in this way can summon the resources necessary to attain them.

Runes: Eihwaz and Dagaz

Two runes offer guidance at the Soul Star Chakra: Eihwaz, the rune of liberation and initiation into the Great Mystery, and Dagaz, the rune of awakening and awareness. Dagaz means "day," and represents the coming of dawn in the physical as well as the spiritual sense. Eihwaz is an invitation to universal mystery, while Dagaz is an invitation to universal wisdom. Both of these runes connect you to the Soul Star Chakra because they activate ascension energies. They are both unembodied runes, meaning that their significance is relevant for the spirit versus the physical body. Use your writing tools to draw these sacred symbols, activating their energy systems and helping bring you into a stronger, more liberated state of consciousness.

Planets: North and South Lunar Nodes

The study of the lunar nodes is sometimes referred to as evolutionary astrology or developmental astrology, because this information illuminates a long path of growth over the course of your soul's most recent incarnations. The North lunar node of the moon shows you which astrological sign represents your deepest soul work in your current lifetime, while the South lunar node represents the astrological sign you embodied in your most recent past life. Once you know where you have been and understand where you are now—and once you integrate the lessons of both—you will be well-prepared to build a strong future.

The Soul Star Chakra represents your ascension in light of this knowledge and wisdom about your soul and your path. For many people, revelations about past and present karma become a powerful impetus for growth, and help the soul evolve more quickly, accelerating spiritual progress. By identifying the house location and sign of your North and South nodes, you will be able to understand your karmic lessons from this lifetime as well as the lifetime immediately preceding this one. In doing so, you can identify patterns of behavior and interaction that serve—and hinder—your spiritual progress.

Archetypes of the Soul Star Chakra

Arguably, the Soul Star Chakra represents *every* archetype, for there is a unique face of the Divine within each archetype. The Soul Star Chakra is the amalgam of all of the faces of the Divine, and so it includes all beings, all archetypes, and all energies in their highest evolutionary form. Think of it as the best of the best.

To anchor this chakra in a material example, though, **The Shaman** comes forward as its archetypal representation. "Shaman" comes from the Siberian word *saman*, or "keeper of knowledge." These days, human beings have a way of taking deep spiritual concepts and processing them through the lens of the intellect (perhaps due to our experience as children of the Industrial Revolution and Scientific Method, who value hard work, facts, and data). Thus, in Western culture, we often look for and privilege education, training, and credentials when we seek someone deeply spiritual. However, there are no credentials in the realm of the spirit, and in many traditions, the wisest elders are also the humblest.

So it is with the archetype of the Shaman, who is the healer in the broadest sense of the word. The Shaman is one who watches, experiences, and translates. The Shaman can, with client permission, embark on a spiritual "journey" experience on behalf of a client without his or her physical presence. Shamans are grounded channels of divine wisdom. They know how to access all of the chakras, how to move within and between them, and how to integrate the wisdom that each one offers. They know how to balance and align the chakras to improve energy flow and function. What's more, they understand the life cycle and have seen all its phases, so they are threshold-keepers who guard the sacred doorways to life and death.

To work with the archetype of The Shaman, set an intention for the integration of all dualities in your life and call upon the four cardinal directions (north, south, east, and west) to be present to you. Then, work closely with the plant, animal, and crystal allies, learning to respect those tools as sacred helpers on your path. The more you attune yourself with nature's cycles and her offerings, the more easily you will ascend to your next level of soul wisdom.

Mantra of the
Soul Star Chakra

In Sanskrit, the mantra of peace is *Om Shanti Om. Om* is the sound of the name of God, and *shanti* means peace in Sanskrit. Together, these words call in the peace of God/Source/Creator energy. Use this beautiful mantra whenever you feel sad or overwhelmed. (It also resonates with children, since it is easy to pronounce and introduces them to two of the most important words in the Sanskrit language.) Open the door to ascension by calling upon the peace of Source. There are levels of peace, and the deepest peace does not come from within—it comes from above. Once you begin to receive this highest level of universal peace, you will have a sense of the interconnectedness of all life. You came to this planet and this life from that oneness, and part of you longs to return to it.

Allow yourself the opportunity to receive this gift of loving union with All That Is: When you attune yourself with the Oneness of All Creation, you recognize yourself as one sacred part of the whole. In this way, you release your need to control, manipulate, or change your life circumstances. Instead, you begin to trust that everything you need is already being provided to you in every moment, and all is well.

Embodiment Exercise:
Soul Star Chakra Activation

To activate the Soul Star Chakra is to take your place among the Children of the Stars. By acknowledging your own sacred nature, you open yourself to receiving wisdom, guidance, and truth, and to connecting with All That Is. You open yourself to connecting with the Oneness of Creation. These are lofty concepts and yet, the purpose of life is to evolve and ascend so that you can reconnect to a deeper sense of unity. Use this meditation to guide you on this path.

1/ Remember that your body has lived one mortal life, but your soul has crossed many lifetimes. Your soul may feel young and energetic or tired and weary. No matter how it feels, honor the beauty of your spirit now. You may do this exercise sitting or lying down in a comfortable resting position. Whichever position you choose, close your eyes and say "thank you" quietly to yourself. You have walked a long road.

2/ Now, extend your gaze skyward (outdoors, if you can) and lift your face to the sun. Open your eyes and your arms wide and feel the air around you, the breeze blowing, and let yourself hear the sounds of nature that embrace you. Be fully in this precious moment.

3/ Then, when you are ready, recite your *Om Shanti Om* mantra aloud. Stretch each word out, fully articulating each syllable, and take a long, deep breath in between each repetition. As you say each word, focus your attention on the meaning behind it. Really sense the presence of God as you say *Om*, and then receive the blessing of peace as you say *Shanti*. Repeat *Om* one last time, and then take a breath. Breathe, repeat; breathe, repeat. Do this for as long as you are called.

4/ Bring your hands together in front of you, folded in prayer pose, and pull them tight in toward your chest, aligned slightly to the left, over your heart. Feel your heart beat against your hands, and give thanks for the blood that flows in your veins. Give thanks for your breath, for your body, and for this life you are blessed to live.

5/ Now, give thanks for your spirit and your wisdom. Give thanks for your connection to the Divine, for the peace you experience, for your spiritual gifts. Give thanks for your ability to trust your intuition and hear the voice of the Divine, for the beauty that surrounds you, and your ability to see the art of the Divine. Give thanks for the many people and beings who love you in this lifetime, and your ability to feel and sense their love.

6/ Gratitude is the key to magic, to ascension, and to peace. As you embody this deep state of peace and ascension, give yourself permission to enjoy this moment. Many spend their whole lives seeking this moment of union and surrender. Allow it to wash over and purify you from within and without. Give thanks to each part of your body and invite yourself to relax and soften as you step further into this state of enlightened bliss.

May your journey be blessed as you ascend toward the Soul Star. Amen, A'ho, So it is. And on we go.

Conclusion: Giving the Chakras a Voice

In this, the final chapter of this book, each chakra is given a voice here to speak to you directly so as to offer its wisdom. These are channeled, high-frequency messages designed to help you connect even more deeply with each of the nine energy centers explored in this book. As you prepare to enjoy each section, take a moment to call your energy into present time, inhale deeply and exhale fully, and consider anointing yourself with one of the essential oils for each of the chakras to help open your other channels of awareness. You could choose to hold one of the gemstones of that chakra as you read; or, perhaps, simply lying down in a comfortable position, wrapped in a warm blanket, feels best to you. Trust and follow your intuition in this (and in all things).

This chapter is not an "intellectual" chapter; it is a spiritual experience of energy concepts translated into the written word. Allow yourself to melt into the words of this chapter. When words are translated through spirit, they take on a different vibration. The words that follow have the capacity to open, heal, restore, soothe, and bless you. Meet them from where you are today, and let them take you where you are intended to go.

Amen, A'ho, So it is. And on we go.

If the Earth Star Chakra Could Speak ...

I would speak to you of deep chambers in the innermost layers of the Earth's core, where all of the ancestors' bones create a pyramid of lived wisdom. This wisdom takes root deep in the Earth and feeds the crystals and minerals as they form over thousands of years. The ancestors speak these words of wisdom through the gem and mineral people, the rock and stone people, and the bone spirits. When you work with rock or bone, you are harnessing stored energy from ages past. You can rest down here in this labyrinth of wisdom and time. Set down your worries and cares and take a seat. Stay for a while—for thousands of years, if you like. This place is not unfamiliar to your spirit, for you have traveled here before. Here your aunts and uncles commune with your great-great-grandparents, who connect to the ones who initiated your line. You are well known here.

When you work with your crystals and minerals, you are working with me, too—Vasundhara, Daughter of the Earth. I am your grandmother, too, the embodied union of your wise woman ancestors across time. Can you hear us? We seek only to comfort and protect you from the cares of this world. We are here to remind you that you truly are held in a womb of love at all times, and you do not need to do or be anything special to deserve or receive this love. It is simply yours now, as it has always been.

If I, the Earth Star Chakra, could speak, I would offer you the blessing of my bountiful and strong embrace. You can place your faith in me, for I am strong enough to hold you and anchor you, to tether you to a place that will not fail or resist you. Here you will never experience rejection or sorrow, for here you are known, seen, held, appreciated, and wanted. Here you are the child that was deeply desired by both of her parents, and here you are the child whose needs are met by a community of loving souls whose ultimate priority is your care and well-being. I see you.

If the Root Chakra Could Speak …

I would speak to you of protection, for mine is the chakra of safety and home. I would want you to understand that safety is your birthright. All sentient creatures care for their young and do so on the basis of instinct, not desire. If you were not cared for in this way, you deserve to find protection now in your adult years, for safety is still your birthright. I am here to take your hand and show you the way. I have many tools I can offer you for this work. You are not doing this work alone; many on this planet right now feel lost and afraid, alone without direction or guidance.

Let me introduce you to the plant and flower kingdom and the many allies you have there. When you work with flowers and flower essences or herbs and essential oils, you are in the realm of the Root Chakra, the borderland between what is visible and what is buried, the present and the past. When you connect with the plant medicines and sacraments that present themselves as healers and messengers of hidden wisdom, you make the spiritual progress necessary for you to fulfill your soul's purpose for incarnation. This work is very important. Take the time to learn the ancient names of familiar herbs, for even their names offer vibrational magic. Touch the herbs and flower petals, rubbing them between your fingers, releasing their sacred essence and perfuming your body and hair with their oils. Enjoy working with the fruits of my trees, the flowers on my vines. They are my art, and I toil over them in anticipation of your joy.

Next, let us walk alongside the spirit animal helpers who have arrived to support us. In the east, birthplace of new beginnings, eagle and condor fly to meet us and help us see our lives from a loftier angle. Jaguar and hummingbird meet us in the south to connect us with fire element energies. We move west to find crow and black bear waiting, patient teachers of insight and integration. Then in the north, all of the snow creatures arrive: deer, bison, moose, buffalo, and elk, with their teachings of process and time, grounding and proud strength.

If I, the Root Chakra, could speak, I would tell you that you never walk alone. Here you walk among giants and ancient ones, beings of stone and light who are patient and all-seeing. Here you are rescued from the struggle of life; you need only say yes and allow us to hold you, sweet one. I see you.

If the Sacral Chakra Could Speak …

I would speak to you of passion and desire, and tell you tales of adventures in longing and lust. I would summon you into my chamber and urge you to leave your hesitations outside, for mine is the chakra of exploration into the secret desires of our hearts. Mine is also the chakra of life, for it is within my womb that life nests, anchors, and grows. My ability to inspire, seduce, and create is the source of my power, and it is not a power to be underestimated.

When you feel disconnected from your inner goddess and your deepest desires, simply call upon me. I am here to remind you of the most delicate aspects of your sensual beauty. I can remind you of the way your eyes glisten in the sun or the beautiful way your hands move when you speak. I will tell you tales of how others have desired you and longed for your attention. I will mirror back to you the many ways you have brought beauty to this world by expanding your capacity to love, to desire, and to create. As the last of the lower chakras, I will anchor your magic in your physical body to keep you grounded and connected as you move and explore the treasures of this world.

When you work with the element of fire, you are activating one of my primary channels for Sacral Chakra energy. Masculine fire energy can fill depleted reserves and strengthen you in times of challenge or confusion. I am the chakra of clarity and motion: As my delegate of this sacred work, the Fire Element will push you forward and offer momentum to stay the course in all you do.

If I, the Sacral Chakra, could speak, I would tell you that you are worthy of desire just as you are right now, today. You are a magnificent vessel of creative potential and every curve of your body is a delight worthy of deep and slow exploration. Your lips spill seductive secrets; your eyes, aglow with the fire burning inside of you, are windows to a soul that has so much living left to do. I am here to whisper in your ear, "Keep going." Your best and sexiest years are ahead, goddess, and a universe of passions awaits you. I see you.

If the Solar Plexus Chakra Could Speak ...

I would speak to you of power, because you have arrived in the human body's epicenter of personal power, self-esteem, ego, and will. Here, in my space, power is not just a concept, but also a currency, a flow of energy you can connect to as you wish. I would tell you stories of power and prestige, tales of conquest

from ancient civilizations—stories of war and bloodshed, but also of sovereignty and divine-right authority bestowed upon humans by God. Many think of power as a curse, but I am here to remind you that power is one of the keys to peace. To find happiness, you must feel as though you can influence the outcomes of your life. The events of your life are not just happening to you; they are happening through you, because of you, and in light of you. You are a divine co-author of your life.

When you work with the sun, you harness the direct energy of my frequency. Allow the warm rays of the sun to penetrate your own energy field and fill you with an overwhelming sense of confidence and purpose. Feel yourself stand taller as you turn your face to the sun and give thanks for the blessings offered to you here. Let yourself rest here, basking in its comforting embrace. In this moment, everything is in order and just as it should be. In this moment, you are capable of all that you desire to create in life. You are powerful, competent, and worthy. You have the skills you need to live this one life to its fullest limits, experiencing every joy and blessing. You have the energy it takes to become your true, authentic self and to express your full essence in the world. Nothing about you needs to be changed, molded, or adapted to suit anyone else's needs.

If I, the Solar Plexus Chakra, could speak, I would tell you to rise, queen. Rise, king. Take your rightful place in the universe as a bright star capable of birthing a universe. You do not take orders from others. You do not bow to another's commands. You are the ruler of your realm, and your sovereignty is unquestioned. Your authority is both legitimate and valuable. You have much to learn, but you also have much to share. The world needs you. May you come to see the power you have always held. I see you.

If the Heart Chakra Could Speak ...

I would speak to you of love, for here in my arms you can find the unconditional tenderness you have sought for many lifetimes. I am here to teach you how to both give and receive love.

Oh, how the heart becomes wounded in this life. Desires mingle with expectations and then the reality of humanity sets in. People can only give so much, love so much, offer so much. There is always a limit in the mortal realm. Humans can only do so much with what they have and where they are. It is not for lack of desire or will—it simply is. You seek a spiritual love—a love that transcends time and space. A love that feels like home. When humans speak of home, connect to the idea of home, they are anchoring themselves in the Universal Home—the star systems from which all of our souls emerged many thousands of years ago to pioneer the human experience on Earth—from which all souls collectively descend and to which all souls return.

If I, the Heart Chakra, could speak, I would remind you that love is truly all there is. You are here to see, experience, learn, give, and receive love. Nothing more, nothing less. My greatest teaching to you, if you can receive it, is that people are flawed and will fail you. You must find a way to love them anyway. Life will bestow hundreds of moments of magic upon you, if you can pause long enough to see and appreciate them. Those moments will sustain you when it seems like all is lost. Let yourself be immersed in those moments and know that more always come. They always come. Love always comes.

Love eludes the human grasp. Cling to it too tightly, and love flees; ignore it too long, and love disappears. Love needs even and consistent care, appreciation, and acknowledgment to flourish. That is the secret: Tell love often that it is loved. In return, love will tell you often that you are loved. Love wants you to experience ease and flow. When you stop struggling, you will float. I promise. I see you.

If the Throat Chakra Could Speak ...

I would speak to you of your voice and your ability to articulate, understand, see, and honor truth. Now is the time for you to step into an authentic way of living and being, because hiding your true self prevents you from making spiritual progress.

When you work with your voice—through speaking, writing, or singing—you make a sacred offering to the universe because your voice is needed. Your message is sacred. Your gifts are unique.

And you were created in the image of the divine to bring these gifts to the planet at this time. You were chosen for a reason.

When you work with the crystals of angelic presence, you connect with me as well, for my chakra is the domain of angels. Here, where your truth lives, so too does the voice of your truth and the fullest expression of your authentic self. When you live deeply, accepting all of yourself—even the parts that seem unlovable—you are presenting a gift to the entire cosmos. Your most powerful guardian angel is, ironically, you. Both power and protection truly come from within. You are both mortal and immortal, and the immortal parts of you keep watch over the mortal parts. That is why protection is your birthright; you carry it with you.

The entire universe seeks to hear your voice. Speak! Sing! Let all who surround you learn the songs of your soul. If you need to yell, yell! Scream and shout, and then laugh, cry, and let it all fall to silence for a moment. Silence can also be a facet of your voice.

If I, the Throat Chakra, could speak, I would tell you that your truth is Truth. You are right where you need to be, doing what you need to do, and your fullest self—with all your flaws—is beautiful. I see you.

If the Third Eye Chakra Could Speak ...

I would speak to you of knowing and wisdom. I would ask you what is troubling you in order to help you interpret the signs presenting themselves to you as occluded symbols and mysteries. I would teach you to see with all three of your eyes—your two human eyes to see, and your one knowing eye to understand.

At the Third Eye Chakra, a new dimensional world becomes available to you. As you inch closer to the border between the physical body and the soul, your awareness begins to drift away from the things of mortal concern and your consciousness expands to include the greater collective of spirits that incarnated together in this lifetime. You are here to help and guide others, as they are here to help and guide you.

When you look outside of yourself for tools to use in helping others, never forget that your greatest tool is your intuition. It speaks a thousand languages and is as old as time. It knows both the masculine and feminine path, and so nothing in the human realm is foreign to your deepest knowing. When you begin to doubt yourself and your access to this knowing, you need to spend more time right here, in this sanctuary of insight. Go within, not without, to find the answers to all of your heart's questions.

If I, the Third Eye Chakra, could speak, I would remind you that you already have the answers to your questions; you may simply not have access to them right now because you are not ready to see. Sometimes the spirit guides are benevolent that way: They bring to your vision and attention only the concepts and realities you are prepared to receive and integrate into your present level of awareness. Begin dialogue with your guides: Ask for signs and wisdom. Ask to be shown what you are ready to receive now. Know that intuition sometimes appears as a series of tiny locked doors. Each tiny door of truth or awareness that you unlock leads you to another. Keys to each door are provided when and as you are ready. Be in a state of gratitude for the many keys you have already been given, and be in a state of trust that more keys are arriving. When the signs come, integrate and act fearlessly upon them. You are always shown what you need to see, even if what you see is difficult for you to accept. Remember that all wisdom is a blessing. In your quest for wisdom and truth, know that I see you.

If the Crown Chakra Could Speak …

I would speak to you of your oneness with Source and divine union, for here at the Crown Chakra you experience for the first time your absolute connection to Source energy. On many levels you know that you are a spiritual being in human form, but it is not until you engage the Crown Chakra that you begin to embody this truth and live it in a way others can see, experience, and learn from.

I would remind you that you are a teacher, and your greatest lesson is love. It has always been love, and will always be love.

It is a challenge to teach love if you have not experienced it yourself. Even without the experience of love in physical form, you are still obliged to learn, embody, and teach love. That is why Crown Chakra work is the hardest of all for some, while it comes naturally and effortlessly for others. How you experience the Crown Chakra is about how your spirit evolves in this lifetime, which is anchored in not just your past on this planet but your past lives as well. At the Crown Chakra, we are reunited with Source/God/Creator as a means of helping us to experience, on a spiritual level, the love we may not have been given on a physical or emotional level. The Crown Chakra fills in the gaps of the Heart Chakra with an even more profound kind of love—one that is unconditional and universally accessible to all.

When you work with sound tools, yoga, and meditation, you are actively opening the channel to receive Crown Chakra energy. Through drumming, breathing, and quieting the mind we find ourselves in an intimate dance with our creator. Crystal and plant allies also offer themselves as points of access to the Great Mystery. The sacred Lakota prayer *Mitakuye Oyasin*, which means "all are related," is a powerful mantra for the Crown Chakra, as it is a central access point for all energies, all levels of consciousness, and all faces of the divine.

If I, the Crown Chakra, could speak, I would urge you to see the entire world as both your mirror and your muse, reflecting your own beauty back to you and inspiring you to become something greater than you are today. I would encourage you to see your own magic in the magic of others, in the tiniest miracles—right down to the unfurling of the smallest leaf on the plants and trees. When the cares of the world feel like too much to witness or carry, remember who you are and more importantly, what you are: an echo of the divine. I bow to the divine in you, and I see you.

If the Soul Star Chakra Could Speak …

I would speak to you of magic beyond your experience or imagination, for here in my realm, time and space collapse in on each other. They support the edges of the third dimension and so they anchor your human reality as you experience it today. Thus, you may not even be able to consciously conceive of what is possible at the Soul Star Chakra. You cannot live in the Soul Star Chakra, but you can reach it. It is available to you. The gestures here, though, must be intentional. Your permission is required.

At the Soul Star Chakra, you will find a peace that is not accessible through the traditional seven-chakra system. Here, peace is not just part of the energy field: It *is* the energy field. Nothing exists outside of peace at the Soul Star Chakra. I see how you struggle with your own process to locate peace and I want to assist you, guide you, teach you. Although you are a teacher, a wise one, a guru to others, you still need to be taught and guided. There is still much you do not know. Much of that mystery resides here, in my domain. Welcome. Your arrival has been planned.

When you work with ascension tools and beings of higher dimensions, you are activating my energy. There are few ascension tools—crystals, candles, herbs, oils—for humans to access at this time, because most people are not doing this work. However, this is not something to mourn or worry about. Not all are ready; in fact, most are not. And yet ascension is the End Game of all incarnations in your universe. When the time comes for ascension work to begin, every aspect of the person's life becomes a tool, and every person in her life becomes a teacher capable of facilitating progress and development. You do not need to seek tools of ascension. When the time arrives, tools and teachers will appear. This is law.

If I, the Soul Star Chakra, could speak, I would remind you of the simplicity and intelligence of all things. Humans have made spiritual matters so complex, but they are natural, equivalent, automatic, and intelligently designed. There is a grand architecture in the universe that you are prevented from seeing, for the sight of it would make human life impossible. How would you continue to agree to struggle through the challenges and toils of this life if you knew that ease and grace were all around you, all the time?

Yet toil you must—at least a little—to learn the lessons and pass the trials. In the universe, there has always been an exchange—a this for a that, a consequence for every action. This law of reciprocity is a basic law of fundamental physics that explains most of the magic you experience as a human—the ebb, the flow. Ascension requires embodiment of the truths of the universe. You are in that process now, and I see you.

Acknowledgments

All beauty begins with a vision. I want to thank my editor, Jill Alexander, who first reached out and made my dream of writing a book a reality. Thank you for bringing your wisdom and magic to this process. I also can't thank Roberta Orpwood enough for creating such incredible watercolor art throughout. Thank you for making this book a feast for the eyes. Editing this book was a joy thanks to the assistance and friendship of Megan Buckley; special thanks also to project editor, Meredith Quinn; art director, Anne Re; everyone who worked behind the scenes to put this book together; and the brilliant duo helping to promote the book and make sure it's available to those who seek it, Erika Heilman and Lydia Anderson. A'ho.

This book would never have been written without the loving support of my Sage Goddess community—both in person and online. Thank you to everyone who has helped me and supported me and the work I do. You know who you are, and I love you. I am here, you are here, we are here. Remember that this book is for you. A'ho and on we go.

My husband and my children are the heart center of my life, and I want you to know that I am so grateful for your presence. This book is also for you. Your love for me, and mine for you, inspired every word written here. I want to thank my parents Nick and Marie, my brother Jeff, my sister Kristin, as well as my soul sister BrookeLynn, my mentors and dearest friends Patty and Leo, Andrew, Carol, Jacque, Sherri, Collin, Denise, Mikyle, Leticia, and all of my beloveds who looked after me, cheered me on, and celebrated milestones with me. A'ho.

Team SG: You are the magic! I work with the most talented people in the world, and each of them brings his or her own unique talents and skills to the work we do, with one mission: To heal the world one gesture at a time. BrookeLynn, Sona, Claire, our photographers, design team, writers, and social media and marketing team. Our production team, our wrap and ship team. Our support and customer care team. Our technical team, our warehouse team. The lovely ladies of the SG showroom. Thank you for the work you do every day to hold the space; thank you for always making sure every customer is seen. I see you and honor you. This book is for you, and my hope is that it will show you a way to work with the many energies you hold in your roles each day. A'ho.

I am a student of life and have been blessed to learn in the company of masters. To my greatest teachers: Dr. Sample, Dr. Bennis, Kathy, Julia, Lorrie, Elaine, John, Christyne, Pixie, Rose: Thank you for breathing the breath of inspiration, confidence, magic, healing, and surrender into me and by extension, into this book. If the words are dense but spacious, enchanting but accurate, deep but resonant, challenging but accessible, it is because you have taught me to be so. You have held those mirrors up to me, and I am ever in your service. A'ho.

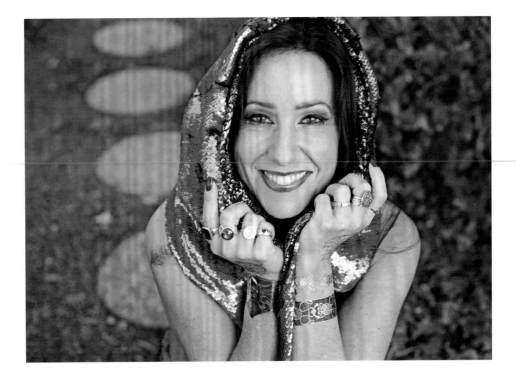

About the Author

Athena Perrakis is the founder and CEO of Sage Goddess, the world's largest source of sacred tools and metaphysical education. She holds a Ph.D. in educational leadership and was a professor and executive coach before she founded Sage Goddess. She blends her training in Shamanism, aromatherapy, Reiki, world history, linguistics, comparative religion, and leadership to bring a perspective that is both theoretical and practical.

Athena feels strongly that all spiritual paths are, in fact, One Path moving in the same direction, working toward the same goals, and anchored in the same history. Her desire to find a common thread and unite the world around their common experiences has inspired many people to connect with their own roots and find healing, forgiveness, and peace. By seeking the presence of Source within and honoring one's own divinity, one effortlessly finds beauty in the world.

The Sage Goddess community on Facebook includes 700,000 fans from around the world who are seeking the path to integrated spirituality. Sage Goddess is headquartered in Los Angeles, California, and has a storefront where visitors can meditate, shop for sacred tools, and experience live ritual each month at the full moon.

About the Illustrator

Roberta Orpwood is a Professional Visionary Artist, Reiki Master Teacher, and Shamanic Sound and Energy Healer who works from her private Studio and Therapy Practice within South West London.

Her delicate watercolor paintings are influenced by her love of natural beauty, the female figure, the spirit of nature, and the mystery of the human soul. Her creations are predominantly figurative, expressing beauty beyond the limits of the physical body. They represent a divine feminine that resides within all of us, and her compositions are often inspired by the visions she receives during her shamanic journeying and meditation practice. They include not only goddesses but spirit animals, guides, elementals, and soul portraits, with themes of love, healing, and empowerment.

www.soulbirdart.com

Index

A

A'HO AND ON WE GO.